Doctor Yourself

Natural Healing That Works

Andrew Saul, Ph.D.

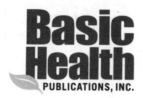

Basic Health
PUBLICATIONS, INC.

Basic Health Publications, Inc.
28812 Top of the World Drive
Laguna Beach, CA 92651
949-715-7327 • www.basichealthpub.com

Library of Congress Cataloging-in-Publication Data
Saul, Andrew W.
    Doctor yourself : natural healing that works / Andrew W. Saul ;
foreword by Abram Hoffer.
        p. cm.
Includes bibliographical references.
    ISBN-13 978-1-59120-033-8
    ISBN-10 1-59120-033-4
    1. Orthomolecular therapy—Popular works. 2. Naturopathy—Popular
works. I. Title.

    RM235.5.S38   2003
    615.8'54—dc21

                                        2003009645

Editor: Rowan Jacobson
Typesetter: Gary A. Rosenberg
Cover design: Mike Stromberg

Printed in the United States of America

10   9   8   7   6   5

Contents

PART TWO: Natural Healing Tools and Techniques

For Michael, Gabriel, and Raphael

*Special thanks to
Helen, Luanne, John, and Richard,
who stood by me regardless*

Foreword

by Abram Hoffer, M.D.

In 1952, when we first began to study the therapeutic properties of vitamin B_3 for the treatment of schizophrenia, my colleagues and I did not think that we were blazing new trails. We merely used much larger amounts of this vitamin than were required to keep anyone free from pellagra. At that time, it was forbidden for medical doctors to have any professional interaction with alternative medicine professions such as homeopathy, chiropractic, and naturopathy. Even sharing an office with them could lead to the financial death of losing one's license to practice. So we happily carried on with our work, gathering more and more data showing how powerful niacin and niacinamide were in helping to treat the schizophrenias, among the worst of all human diseases.

We were rudely awakened when we began to publish our findings in the psychiatric literature. To my surprise, I discovered that our conclusions were not accepted with grace and interest. They were rejected with boredom, or hostility and anger. At the time I was both a professor of psychiatry and director of psychiatric research. But because of the vitamin research I was doing, I was in an awkward situation. I could not be politically loyal to the medical school and to the profession of psychiatry if I continued to advocate megadoses of niacin. I chose to give my loyalty to my patients.

Gradually, a few brave physicians, mostly American psychiatrists previously trained as analysts, began to use the treatment we had described and slowly we began to make some headway. The medical associations fought us tooth and nail every step of the way, but interest in our work continued to grow. We were far from the first to point out the importance of good food, but we were the first to show that very large "megadoses" of some vitamins were therapeutic when usual vitamin doses were not. (Actually, the first controlled experiment that showed the importance of good food was published in the Bible, in the first chapter of the Book of Daniel. It was an open study.)

Today, orthomolecular medicine is beginning to flourish. "Orthomolecular" means using a therapeutic substance that is natural to the human body, such as a vitamin or mineral. There has been a major paradigm shift away from the "old school," which maintained that a few easy dietary rules as promoted by governments and medical associations would ensure everyone's good health. Every year, more and more authors join the orthomolecular field, publishing good books that set the record straight about vitamins and put power into the hands of patients.

Doctor Yourself is one of these. In it, the reader will find information on a large number of conditions, ranging from attention deficit disorder in children to Alzheimer's, arthritis, women's health issues, alcoholism, cancer, diabetes, the problems with vaccination, and many more. As Dr. Saul shows, all of these conditions are treatable through natural means. In fact, they are best treated that way.

It is high time somebody said this, because natural means have been almost totally ignored. The body is composed of innumerable molecules developed over billions of years by the toughest test of all: survival. We are finely tuned organisms, with a dizzying number of different compounds and reactions. To think that one can insert a strange molecule that has never before been there, and hope to correct some malfunction, is the height of folly. The only molecules that are therapeutic are orthomolecular ones—those that are normally present and with which the body is familiar. I can't think of a single toxic molecule that has ever truly cured anything. The only compounds that have been used successfully in chronic ailments are the nutrients, vitamins, minerals, amino acid, essential fatty acids, and hormones. And when one tries to replace natural hormones by compounds that are slightly different in order to have patent protection, the results are dismal.

By writing this foreword, I mean to give Dr. Saul, and the other writers in this field, the recognition and honor due to them for preparing for the eventual takeover of all health care by safe, effective nutritional medicine. *Doctor Yourself* represents a new type of comprehensive medical reference book. With this book, Dr. Saul is making a major contribution toward consolidating what is known in the huge and growing field of natural, orthomolecular medicine. Some day it will be considered malpractice for any healer anywhere to ignore the vast importance of nutrition and the optimum use of nutrients in preventing and healing disease, as is detailed in this book. I urge all readers to promote *Doctor Yourself* to their physicians. Some of them will be grateful.

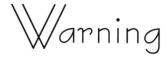Warning

Do Not Read This Page

In fact, do not read this book. Put it back right now, because you are only going to get into trouble for reading it. Your family, your doctor, your professor, your druggist, your newscaster, your TV set, and your undertaker will all oppose what you'll learn inside here: how to get healthy, naturally, and affordably.

As a teacher for some years, I found that most folks never read the instructions on a test (or on anything else, for that matter). You could label a part of any exam INSTRUCTIONS and then you could put all the answers right there, safe in the knowledge that no one would see a single one.

Well, now you've done it. You are still holding my book even after all this. Glad to have you aboard, but don't say I didn't warn you.

And about those answers: please read "How to Use This Book" for a jump start on getting yourself well.

How to Use This Book

1. You can look up an illness in the Contents or Index, or

2. You can read the book straight through because I am such a witty and fascinating writer, or

3. You can read it straight through for a holistic picture of a natural lifestyle, and then make your own overall healthy lifestyle changes.

Nobody is interested in vitamins. For that matter, nobody is all that whooped up about health. What people want to know is how to cure disease. This goes for preoccupied doctors as much as for desperate patients. In more than twenty-five years of lecturing on natural health care, I have almost never had anyone come up to me afterward and say, "Tell me more about the biochemistry of vitamin therapy." Rather, the ubiquitous follow-up question is, "What vitamins should I use for (such and such an illness)?"

This book is not about vitamins; it is about diseases treatable with vitamins. It is also about any number of other ways in which you can, as I say, "fire your doctor." Should you ever want to put someone to sleep, just start lecturing on nutrition with the ever-boring "vitamins A through E and foods that contain them" approach. I guarantee that heads will be nodding long before you finish with the B complex.

I hope this book, and the bibliography at the close of it, proves useful to patients who are struggling upstream to convince their pharmophilic (drug-lovin') physicians to at least give vitamin therapy the time of day. There is nothing quite like pulling out a whole pile of medical references to shorten physicians' "supplements might hurt you so just eat a good diet" speeches. Even the most ostrichlike orthodox practitioner cannot long resist the call of the peer-reviewed journal reference.

For a real blast of information, trot out Dr. Melvyn Werbach's *Textbook of Nutritional Medicine* and Linus Pauling's *How to Live Longer and Feel Better* next time somebody tries to tell you that more research is needed before vitamins can be used to treat illness.

Still, there remains the real possibility that your doctor will recoil when presented with all these references. This reaction, true to human nature, is nevertheless unscientific. It is embarrassing to doctors when patients know more about their case than they do. Yet there is no other rational choice. If therapy exists, and is reasonably well-tested and safe, it is inexcusable not to try it. Doctors know this, but are so uneducated on nutrition that they are usually not in a position to supervise such therapy. Hence the embarrassment. Let us, therefore, provide the continuing education they so sorely need.

Obviously, you need to do some reading first, but you do not have to read it all. Do you read the dictionary cover to cover? (You don't have to, because, as comic Steven Wright says, "The zebra did it.") Just look up the diseases that are closest to home.

Most people pick up health books because they want immediate information about a disease, either their own or that of a loved one. So *Doctor Yourself* presents many protocols (instructions) for the natural treatment of illnesses. The balance of the book consists of personal experiences and case stories. I like writing these the best.

There are immediate objections to such a book, and they include the following:

1. **"The author is not a physician."** And I'm not, believe me. Physicians often write strikingly weak health books. I have looked through many doctor-authored books on arthritis, heart disease, fertility, ADHD, allergies, and countless other topics without finding any serious consideration of natural healing or therapeutic nutrition. These doctors, and therefore the public, are largely unaware of the proven value of natural healing in treating serious disease. *Doctor Yourself* contains enough scientific references that a reader will either say, "Wow, this is it!" or, "They are all liars . . . liars by the hundreds." I think the public is tired of medication, and ready for education. If delivered with style, we will read.

   To misquote one Dr. Leonard McCoy: "Damn it, Jim, I'm a teacher, not a doctor!" I do not prescribe, I describe. People need alternative health information. Here's some good stuff. What you do with it is up to you.

2. **"There are health books like this on the market already."** And good ones, too. My bibliography lists dozens and dozens. So go ahead: put this book down and go read them.

   One reason you may not jump to do that is because even the best natural health books share a common fault. Most are fine references, but make for dry reading. Not *Doctor Yourself.* You are going to like this one. Though I hardly understand why, my writing has been described as "outrageous," among other epithets. You may coin a few of your own before you're through.

   Health self-help books should be fun to read. Most of the best scientific natural therapeutics information has not reached the people who need it most because it's too hard to understand. People need health research presented for them the way a sports announcer describes a ball game. That's what I try to do. At the same time, a health book needs to be full of practical how-to techniques, backed by specific medical references, and to be based on considerable experience. You'll get plenty of that here. As a college lecturer, I liked to rock the scientific boat, trotting out study after study showing proven natural alternatives to pharmaceutical medicine.

3. ***"Hey, where's my illness?"*** If you searched the Contents and Index and did not find the topic you're looking for, you might suppose that perhaps this book is not for you. There are thousands of illnesses. You know I cannot cover them all. Plus, your arms are not strong enough to carry home the library big enough to present all knowledge of all healing of all ailments. While it has been my experience that most people like an "organized by illness" format, a fundamental natural-healing premise is "treat the person, not the disease." This means that there is a lot of topic overlap in *Doctor Yourself,* and that information applicable to one illness may be extended to another. More generally, diet and lifestyle changes benefit a broad spectrum of chronic illnesses. If you live, breathe, and know anyone who ever gets sick, this book is for you.

I offer my readers what I've learned, tried and verified in preventing and also treating real illnesses with safe, inexpensive, and effective drugless techniques. I have been very satisfied with the science behind, and the results gained, with natural healing.

My own kids made it all the way into college and never, not once ever, had a single dose of any antibiotic. One television interviewer told me that this was the best lead-in she had ever had for a guest.

And the best part of it is that it's true.

The Doctor Yourself
Laws of Natural Therapeutics

People often want to know where I'm coming from. After all, some will say, "If this natural healing stuff was so good, my doctor would already have told me about it." My college students frequently wondered why the content of my lectures was so "different" from their other health classes. And certainly all readers of this book deserve to know, up front, just which garden path I am going to lead them down. Fair enough. Here are my "Laws of Natural Therapeutics":

LAW: Most illness is due to malnutrition. This not only includes the chronic diseases, but also viral and bacterial acute illnesses, which are greatly aggravated by inadequate nutrition.

LAW: Adding drugs to a sick body to cure it is like adding poison to a polluted lake to clean it. Killing microorganisms, or masking the cause of symptoms, is no more than a temporary answer.

LAW: Restoring health must be done nutritionally, not pharmacologically. All cells in all persons are made exclusively from what we drink and eat. Neither the chemical spraying of a sick plant nor the chemical dosing of a sick child can substitute for really good nutrition.

LAW: Nutrient therapy increases individual resistance to disease. Drug therapy generally lowers resistance to disease. Healthy plants, healthy animals, and healthy people do not get sick. Doctors do not admit to this, because healthy people make poor customers. What if word got out?

LAW: With vitamin therapy, speed of recovery is proportional to the dosage given. As there is a certain, large amount of fuel needed to launch an aircraft, there is a certain, large amount of nutrients needed to cure a sick body.

LAW: The quantity of a nutritional supplement that cures an illness indicates the patient's degree of deficiency. It is therefore not a megadose of the vitamin, but rather a megadeficiency of the nutrient that we are dealing with.

LAW: Vitamin C can replace antibiotics, antihistamines, antipyretics, antitoxins, and antiviral drugs at saturation (bowel tolerance) levels. "Saturation" means vastly higher doses than you ever imagined, and "bowel tolerance" means exactly what you think it means.

LAW: The reason one nutrient can cure so many different illnesses is because a deficiency of one nutrient can cause many different illnesses.

LAW: A vitamin can act as a drug, but a drug can never act as a vitamin.

LAW: With vitamin therapy, at any given quantity, frequently divided doses are more effective. This is especially true with the water-soluble B and C vitamins.

LAW: Generally, the price of a food is inversely proportional to its nutritional value. Brown rice, beans, vegetables from your garden, sprouts from your own countertop jars, fruits from your own trees and bushes . . . all are superior to meats and prepared convenience foods that cost a fortune.

LAW: What you need to do to doctor yourself is less than you might think but more than you might want. There are no free rides in life.

LAW: Health recovered is proportional to effort expended. You do not have to live an inflexibly perfect life to have a much healthier body . . . but it sure helps to try.

LAW: Most confusion over what constitutes proper health care arises from partisans. Bias against vitamin supplements proceeds from people who stand to lose when cheap, natural health care succeeds. Hospitals, physicians, nurses, dieticians, politicians, pharmaceutical companies, and others have a vested interest in disease.

LAW: Many conflicting reports about vitamin therapy come from natural health partisans. These include vitamin distributors, individual supplement companies, brands, and even practitioners trying to corner as much of the market as they can for themselves. Ignore them. I have no financial connection whatsoever to the health products industry or to any part of it.

LAW: Health knowledge worth having does not go out of date in ten years or even one hundred years. "New" does not automatically mean more accurate or more valuable. "Old" research and clinical studies are often superior references. What works is never out of date. Fasting, near-vegetarian diet, use of nutritional supplements, and other non-pharmaceutical methods have stood the test of time, as have Einstein's theories and the Bill of Rights.

Fire Your Doctor!

If you want something done right, you have to do it yourself. This especially applies to your health care.

I fired my first doctor when I was fifteen. I was away at school and experiencing some anxiety symptoms. Without hesitation and without explanation, the school physician gave me a little white envelope containing half a dozen little green capsules. Before leaving the infirmary, I took two of them, as directed. By the time I got to the campus dining hall, I was higher than a kite. I still remember walking over to the table by the window where my roommate and best friend, Dean, always sat. As I approached, he looked at me quizzically. Me, I just smiled. And I mean all I did was smile. Everything was absolutely, positively fine; there are no worries when you are as heavily doped up as I was. Of course, I could do nothing *but* smile in that state. I did not care if I ate and I do not remember if I did; I had no interest in schoolwork, conversation, or anything else, either. Those little green capsules turned out to contain a very powerful tranquilizer.

It was odd, really, for the year was 1970, and seemingly every student I knew (except Dean and me) was perpetually in search of any way at all to purchase the kind of high I had just received legally, entirely paid for by health insurance, and dispensed from the wise hands of the good ol' school doc.

I never took a second dose of that tranquilizer. Maybe this is because I was a straight-laced good boy. Maybe. More likely, though, the real reason was because I wanted a healthy life. This was a major realization, a truly big step: I realized that the doctor's treatment was seriously amiss. I never went back to the infirmary.

Firing a doctor need not assume the conventional image of a pink slip and a bootprint on the keester. Rather, to fire your doctor means to not need him, to outgrow her, to decide that the doctor's information is incomplete or wrong, and to determine his skill to be insufficient to bet your life on.

To fire your doctor is to hire yourself as your chief physician.

You probably think you are not up to the job. After all, who are you? You didn't go to medical school. That's true, of course. Neither did I. But consider what the limitations of "medicine" are. Drugs and surgical treatments have always been the focus of medical school. Any physician will confirm that, even today, the rest of the curriculum runs far, far behind. Ask your doctor how many courses in clinical nutrition she has completed. Ask you doctor how many hours of homeopathic medicine, herbal medicine, and orthomolecular medicine he has logged. You are likely to find that those "medicines" aren't even counted worthy of time in the medical school syllabus.

Big mistake. Homeopathy has been successfully practiced by physicians the world over for two hundred years. Homeopaths were giving tiny, nontoxic amounts of natural substances to effect a cure while "regular" doctors were drugging people to a premature death with stiff quantities of arsenic and mercury. Herbal medicine goes back for centuries, when practitioners (mostly women) used plants to heal instead of taking blood by the quart from the arms of anybody unfortunate enough to come within the reach of a surgeon's lancet. If anything, drug-and-cut "medicine" is an alternative to the natural health disciplines—and not a very good alternative at that.

And orthomolecular (megavitamin) medicine? There are tens of thousands of references to support it. I have over 4,000 at my DoctorYourself.com website alone. Can all of those successful vitamin-study authors, all those researchers and physicians, be dumber than the reporter you have heard intone that "vitamins may be dangerous and just give you expensive urine"?

Of course not. And far-thinking doctors are beginning to come around to what they were initially taught, and then taught to forget: *vis medicatrix naturae:* the healing power of nature. They have been led back to this timeless principle by their patients, the majority of which see a natural-health practitioner at least once in a given year. The market favors success, and savvy doctors can see the handwriting on the wall.

So now we have the drug physicians trying to learn "natural health," which they want to call "complementary medicine" to keep it in their shop. Monopolistic concerns aside, we should focus on this point: your doctor probably doesn't know any more about natural healing than you do . . . and is likely to know a good deal less. It is a fair race when all parties start at the same time and place. You can learn whatever your doctor learns, just as fast and just as well. You even have several advantages:

First, you have the Home Team Advantage. Your body is better known to you than Yankee Stadium was to Babe Ruth. You live inside you every minute of every day. You can better monitor and adjust your needs than can anyone else.

Second, you only have to learn what you and your family specifically need to know. You have to study up on your own particular health problems, but you do not have to spend time learning about everyone else's. This makes you a specialist in the same time it will make your new study-buddy doctor a poor generalist.

Third, you have the personal, altruistic advantage: you are doing this for your family. Unlike the doctor, you are working for love and life, not money.

Together, these make one tough starting lineup. This is a very powerful, healthy combination, and it will serve you well.

Hire Your Doctor

Now that you have fired your doctor and taken charge of your own health care, it is the perfect time to hire him back. After all, just like a roofer or a plumber, he can be useful for certain things. But, as with those professions, whenever you consult him, remember that your doctor works for you and not the other way around. It is your body. You run the show; your doctor is a subcontractor.

In order for this to work, you need to be on an equal footing with your physician. This is where a lot of people balk and are more than willing to sit down, shut up, and behave. To be on a level playing field with your doctor, first you need to read. Knowledge is power. Read like mad about your condition and the alternatives available for it. Search the library and search the Internet, and do not rest until you have the references to back yourself up.

Next, you need to have a workable physician. If your doctor is not providing you with the care you want, there are two possibilities. One: you have a miscommunication, meaning you have not made it sufficiently clear to your doctor what you do in fact want. Two: you have a disagreement, meaning you have made it clear all right, and the physician is not cooperating with you.

Both of these problems are common, though it is far easier to clear up a miscommunication than a disagreement. I am not saying that you should jettison every doctor that does not knuckle under, but you simply must have a baseline agreement, or any attempts to share information will be futile.

Even polite, personable doctors can still be very paternalistic, sweetly telling you to leave the complicated stuff to them. Hogwash. I would not accept that phrase from a mechanic, plumber, or politician. Neither should you, and in this case your life depends on it. Pleasant office or bedside manner is no substitute for thoroughness.

Do not accept vagueness, either. Nail down a deal, and get your doctor to clearly and unequivocally state his or her acceptance of your wishes. There is no excuse for not trying alternatives with a physician as your copilot. Herbs and vitamins are not perfect, but they are a million times safer than drugs.

With these goals in mind, I offer the following checklist to help you modify and improve the doctor you choose:

Ten Ways to Make Your Doctor into a Naturopath

1. *Pick a workable doctor.* How do you know if a doctor is workable? Interview them. I screen any physician I'm thinking of consulting with. Since there may actually be a charge for this "initial consultation," I carry this out by asking the office manager, nurse or assistant to please relay these three questions to the doctor: (1) "I take vitamin supplements. How do you feel about that?" (2) "I feel that my doctor should work with me, but that I am in charge of my health. Is this compatible with your philosophy of care?" (3) "I choose to decline immunizations. Are you

5

willing to accept this viewpoint?" If the doctor agrees to all three position statements, you are in business. If not, keep looking. Be prepared to spend some time on this process. It pays off.

2. *Not all doctors that promote themselves as "holistic," "alternative," or "complementary" will be as advertised.* Lip service to a natural philosophy is not the same as actually prescribing a fast for obesity or treating pneumonia with vitamin C. Hiring a doctor requires an in-depth evaluation that only personal experience can provide. Word of mouth is a way to capitalize on others' experience with this doctor. Ask around.

3. *Make it easy for your doctor.* Stay healthy. Eat right. Do not smoke. Avoid alcohol and illegal drugs. Keep fit. Show that you take care of yourself.

4. *Do your homework.* Prepare your case before you go in for an office visit. Look up your ailment in the *Merck Manual* to learn what the conventional medical approach to such an illness is. Then read up on the alternatives. You might start with the sizable bibliography at the end of this book. There is no substitute for being well informed.

5. *If you need a diagnosis, get one.* Be responsible. Use technology. Listen to what your doctor has to say, but do not *do* it until you complete step 4, above.

6. *Use the "suggestive selling" technique.* Suggest a natural alternative to any medical treatment you may be offered. Or, instead of one or the other, suggest both. Know what you want and see that you get it.

7. *Look at your situation from the doctor's perspective.* If you were legally bound and professionally constrained to the extent that most physicians are, how would you react to a know-it-all upstart patient who marched into your office and began to dictate terms? To not create a defensive physician, avoid backing your doctor into any corners. Instead, bring along materials written by other physicians who treat naturally. If such-and-such a doctor already does it successfully, it takes the pressure off your doctor in trying it with you. Ask for a "therapeutic trial."

8. *Try the good cop, bad cop approach.* Offer to sign a paper stating that you will not sue the doctor if the natural treatment you request is unsuccessful. At the same time, subtly point out that a patient could sue if the doctor refused a patient's natural treatment request.

9. *Compromise.* Half a pie is better than none. Your doctor does not have to meet you 100 percent on every issue. It is generally sufficient to hear any of the following phrases, which indicate an open-minded physician:

"Vitamins aren't likely to do you any harm."

"I've heard of more and more people doing this."

"I attended a seminar on this recently."

"Let's try it."

"Let me know how this works out for you."

"I told my other patients about this."

10. *Provide positive feedback.* Doctors love to be told that "their" therapy is successful. Whenever appropriate, tell your doctor that you are feeling great. You are likely to be rewarded with, "Whatever you are doing, keep doing it." That is the sweet sound of self-reliant success.

Your Money or Your Health?

As should already be clear, making pharmaceuticals available to everyone won't solve our disease problem any more than making guns available to everyone will solve our crime problem. More vaccinations will do little for the cardiovascular diseases that are responsible for one half of all deaths in the United States. At least half of all illnesses are avoidable, being entirely due to unhealthy lifestyles and eating habits. Only lip service has been paid to preventive medicine, even though America's chronic-or-crisis style of medicine is the very trillion-dollar-per-year boondoggle that got us into this mess in the first place.

I feel very strongly that there is an alternative, a nutritional "road less traveled" that we should have taken long before this. That road is the one of personal responsibility for health, complete dietary overhaul, and, when needed, aggressive high-dose vitamin therapy in place of drugs. The closest professional description of this approach is naturopathy, the organized science of natural healing. There is still time to reverse our steps and take this other path. I perceive a keen need for a direct appeal to individual doctors, students, and patients to improve their health by changing their own lives.

It will not be easy, however. I have personally known more than one physician who was run out of New York State by his peers for practicing naturopathy. This is not a new phenomenon. Since the nineteenth century, the AMA and its clones have declared war on their competitors, eager for a monopoly of the lucrative health field. Has it worked? You decide. One of my most-asked readers' questions remains, "Can you tell me where I can find a natural-healing physician near where I live?"

America's expensive and ineffective healthcare system is fundamentally unworkable. Even the most creative of financial makeovers will not save it. Merely by avoiding megavitamin therapies and downplaying vegetarian diet, it is doomed. Merely by assigning our health responsibility to someone else rather than to ourselves, it is doomed again. The only way to have health care for all individuals is for all individuals to take responsibility for their own health. People need specific instruction on how exactly to do this, and they have not been getting it.

7

Can You Help Me Find a Naturally Minded Physician?

Yes, I can: Look in a mirror.

That's not what you wanted to hear, of course, but that is my answer. Just substituting one doctor for another does not make you self-reliant. It does the opposite: it makes you dependent.

Statements like that tend to bring on more questions, like these: "Doctor myself? Do you honestly think I can become my own doctor?"

Very often, yes. Healing is too big a topic for any one person to know it all. While that statement includes you and me, it also includes your doctor. But it is quite possible to learn more than your doctor knows, particularly in key areas. You may well discover material that your doctor never saw, or did see and never investigated. With a good bibliography, an inquiring mind, and gradual experience, there is no reason why you cannot gain considerable competence in treating yourself and your immediate family in many instances. Remember that in doing your research you will also learn when you really do need a physician.

"Easy to say; hard to do. What if we do it ourselves, and do it wrong?"

I think it is a distinguishing feature of natural therapies that they are straightforward enough and reliable enough to safely do on your own, at home. Medicine has to be dispensed by a pharmacist, surgery by surgeons, drugs by prescription. This is the clearest possible evidence that drug and surgery treatments are inherently unsafe.

"Surely doctors today have far more open minds about alternative health methods."

Medical doctors are called medical doctors for a reason. They go to schools of medicine and they learn medicine and practice medicine. Now substitute the word "nutrition" for the word "medicine" in that sentence and see how impossible it sounds. Most medical personnel remain largely unfamiliar with

Most of what we do to our bodies we do ourselves, daily, by the lifestyle choices we make. There is no outside enemy to fight. We do not need "further study" on mineral and vitamin therapy. The work has already been done, the results are in print, and the public is cheerfully ignorant. How did we miss it?

One possible explanation is the cozy relationship between mainstream medicine and the media. There is more than a hint of collusion. Major wire services are continually fed articles reflecting the positions of the largest, most vocal, and best funded health lobbies and professional trade groups. What is politically correct, popular, and easily reduced to a sound byte is what gets publicity. What gets publicity tends to get funded, and what is funded gets done. Medical witch hunts for a test-tube, magic-bullet cure for cancer or AIDS fit this description. Since pharmaceutical industry investment in such projects is very high, there is funding. Media cooperation is equally high, for a heroic, new celebrity-style medical crusade easily sells papers and commercial air time. On top of that, the American Medical Association has the biggest-spending professional lobby in the country. Politicians know a bandwagon when they see it, and the result is more laws favoring orthodox medicine . . . and still more funding.

non-medical treatments, and tend to dismiss them often without knowing about what they're dismissing. This takes nothing away from their dedication as individuals, but being individuals, they are prone to following certain theories over other theories, favoring particular practices over other alternatives, and holding opinions as often as facts. So it is our responsibility to cover all possible ground in our efforts to cure and prevent illness. If we learn more than the doctor in areas of value to our health, it is our duty to apply this knowledge to the betterment of our family and ourselves. We need total health more than medically approved health. Our wellness should not be limited to our doctor's experience, but enhanced by our own experience.

I believe that your doctor works for you, not the other way around. Your physician is your contractor, and it's your jobsite. Natural therapies aren't just another way to minimize illness but are often a superior way to eliminate illness. Natural healing gets down to the real basics such as your diet and everyday lifestyle—the things that really make us sick, and are really difficult to change. Nature cure is so understandable yet all-embracing that it is best carried out by the patient in daily life. No one can follow you around to see that you eat right, exercise, and live happily. You have to do it yourself.

"If nature cure is so effective, why have my doctors not prescribed it for me?"

It's unreasonable to expect medical doctors and pharmaceutical companies to tell you how to avoid their services by trying the alternatives. You are not going to get a Republican politician to tell you to vote Democratic, and you can't get chow mein in a French restaurant. Hospitals, doctors, and pharmaceutical companies all share a common Achilles' heel: they all profit from disease. I wish this were not the case, but follow the money and consider the results.

"What is the safety of all this?"

Self-care means accepting some risk, and accepting much responsibility. It is not for all people or for all cases. On the other hand, turning over your health to a physician or hospital also involves considerable risk. You have to intelligently chart your own course. Self-care has been highly effective for my family. My kids made it all the way into college without ever having even one dose of any antibiotic. Looking back, I can better see why. This book tells you how. It is up to you do decide what, and when.

9

Considering the paucity of interest (and funding), it is quite remarkable how much good nutrition research has been done, and how almost all of it points to three embarrassingly simple conclusions:

1. The average American's diet is truly terrible, being superabundant in chemicals, calories, and animal protein and very deficient in fiber and diverse major vitamins and minerals.

2. Higher U.S. Recommended Dietary Allowances, plus nutritional supplements, are clearly needed, and even modest increases in vitamin and mineral intake regularly result in both disease prevention and clinical cure.

3. Most citizens, and their doctors, are vaguely aware of item 1, unaware of item 2, and not concerned enough to act on either.

I continue to be amazed at the number of people who actually do not know that huge doses of vitamin C can safely be used as an antibiotic, antiviral, and antihistamine.

Most surprising is the nutritional misinformation level among doctors, who ought to read their own journals but apparently don't. Busy physicians tend to rely on the sales force from pharmaceutical houses the way TV viewers rely on news anchorpersons: just give us the summary. Patent drug companies make money from patented drugs, not generic vitamins. There is much more money to be made with Prednisone than with pyridoxine (vitamin B_6). Doctors' prescriptions generate patent drug sales without the doctor having to pay a cent. Whether nutrition disinterest results from a lack of financial interest, a lack of political clout, or a lack of inclination, the end product is the same: patients are the losers.

My purpose is to help correct this problem by placing both the facts and the motivation directly into your hands. From that point, it is up to you to live healthfully using all available tools to do so. Thorough knowledge of megavitamin nutrition mixed with our own keen need for personal health improvement is such a combustible mixture that a single, well-placed spark will start a good fire. To help provide that initial spark, I have written this book, which blends personal conviction, motivation, and all-too-seldom-seen scientific literature into a guide for students and patients. This project has evolved over nearly thirty years of classroom teaching and private practice as a naturopathic educator.

In the sixties, one slogan was "What if they gave a war, and nobody came?" Enough individual actions could add up to peace. Well, what if each person eats right, exercises, eradicates bad habits, and starts taking vitamins? Might our new slogan be: "What if they gave everybody health insurance, and nobody needed it?" The result would be nothing less than total national health, gained one person at a time.

Oddly enough, it may be that we've had trouble seeing the trees because of the forest. Health care is such an enormous issue that we tend to bite off more than we can chew. Getting a nation to be healthy is one tall order. To think we can ever gain national health by refinancing the same old disease model is ludicrous.

As difficult as it truly is to change our own personal habits, it remains the only sure method to gain back our health, and to positively influence another person to do the same. This book is really about education and motivation in just one person's health behavior, and that is yours.

In the end, education may be reduced to an option, and motivation may be reduced to an offer: there is a way out, and you are free to try it. Many of the lifeboats on the *Titanic* were launched when less than half full. There was a way for hundreds more to be saved, but only for those who 1) knew early that the ship was sinking, and 2) climbed into a boat. Too many of those lost never knew their options until it was too late.

Today, Americans have real health options but are largely unaware of the safety, the scientific validity, and the real curative power of simple nutrients. I have written this book to help people make the discovery, on their own, that there is a way off the sinking ship of conventional drug-and-surgery disease care. That small lifeboat, no matter how flimsy it looks, is a better bet than staying on any big, solid, doomed ship.

Part One

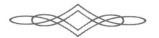

Natural Healing Protocols

The solution to a problem is not always found at the level of the problem. Chasing symptoms can be a dead-end street unless your goal is to personally enrich the stockholders of pharmaceutical companies.

If you suffer from acid reflux or a hiatus hernia, you might want to give these ideas a try.

1. **Make your midday meal your largest**, and do not eat at all after 5 P.M. It is amazing how many indigestion symptoms go away when you do so.

2. **Chew your food very thoroughly.** This sounds too simple to work, so a lot of folks ignore it and miss the benefits. Don't be one of them.

3. **Eat easily digestible food.** This includes fruits, rice, steamed vegetables, sprouted seeds and grains, well-cooked beans, aged cheeses, yogurt, cottage cheese, and *especially* vegetable juices. Avoid fried food. Stop eating meat. (And if you can't manage that completely, at least avoid the worst offenders: cold cuts, ham, pastrami, and pepperoni.)

4. **Try multiple-digestive enzyme tablets**, particularly if you did not follow the advice in step 2, above.

5. Better yet, **eat lots of figs, pineapples, kiwis, mangoes, and papayas**. These fruits are simply loaded with natural digestive enzymes that do half the work for you. *These fruits must be fresh, not canned.* That's because the digestive enzymes are destroyed by cooking temperatures. Dried fruits processed at low temperatures may be okay. A simple way is to try and see.

6. You might also want to up your consumption of good-quality **yogurt**, which contains beneficial digestive bacteria. Make sure you buy a brand that lists live cultures on the label. An old trick from India is to dilute the yogurt in an equal amount of water. This makes it even easier to digest and reduces nose stuffiness.

7. **Raise your head at night.** Sleep on a thicker pillow, or stack up two thin ones. Some people prefer a foam rubber, wedge-shaped bolster pillow.

8. **Chiropractic adjustments** may help. Try three visits and see.

9. **Try the homeopathic remedy (and Schuessler cell salt) Natrum Phos 6X.**

10. **Reduce stress.** Yeah, right! Easier said than done. But the truth is, medi-

tation, relaxation, massage, music, reading, or just some plain old time alone can really make a difference. (Please see my chapter "Stress Reduction.")

11. If your symptoms are really troublesome, **see your physician.** While you are waiting for the appointment, you could go on a vegetable-juice-only diet for three to seven days. Many an appointment has been cancelled by a juice fast.

12. That includes even some serious cases. I have met people who had acid reflux for so long that there was scarring of the esophagus. I acquainted them with the **four-glasses-of-cabbage-juice-a-day** hospital-tested protocol of Garnett Cheney, M.D. While originally used primarily on stomach and lower gastrointestinal conditions, cabbage juice proved effective above the tummy as well. Dr. Cheney found that the entire gastrointestinal tract, from throat to colon, benefits from fresh raw cabbage juice, taken regularly and in quantity. His articles are far from new, but what has changed about cabbage?

Recommended Reading

Cheney G. Antipeptic ulcer dietary factor. *American Dietetics Association* 26 (1950): 9.

Cheney G. The Nature of the antipeptic ulcer dietary factor. *Stanford Medical Bulletin* 8 (1950): 144.

Cheney G. Prevention of histamine-induced peptic ulcers by diet. *Stanford Medical Bulletin* 6 (1948): 334.

Cheney G. Rapid healing of peptic ulcers in patients receiving fresh cabbage juice. *California Medicine* 70 (1949): 10.

Cheney G. Vitamin U therapy of peptic ulcer. *California Medicine* 77, no. 4 (1952).

Nutritional supplements have been used, with considerable success, to help overcome learning disabilities in children. In a well-designed clinical trial, megadoses of vitamins were seen to be safe and remarkably effective, even offering improvement in Down's syndrome children.

Dr. Ruth F. Harrell and associates published their important findings in *Proceedings of the National Academy of Sciences*—in 1981! Although *Medical Tribune* picked the story up, your doctor is likely as unaware of this research as I was until one of my chiropractic students showed it to me in 1993.

What worked then works now.

The Harrell study was successful because her team gave learning-disabled kids much larger doses of vitamins than other researchers: over 100 times the *adult* (not child's) RDA for riboflavin; 37 times the RDA for niacin (given as niacinamide); 40 times the RDA for vitamin E; and 150 times the RDA for thiamine. These are the quantities that evidently get results, and get them safely. Safety and effectiveness are the rule, not the exception, with therapeutic nutrition. I urge you to read the full paper: Harrell RF, Capp RH, Davis DR, Peerless J, and Ravitz LR. Can nutritional supplements help mentally retarded children? An exploratory study. *Proc Natl Acad Sci USA* 78 (1981): 574–8.

Dr. Harrell, who had been publishing on vitamin effects on learning for over thirty years, was not inventing the idea of megavitamin therapy in one paper. Psychiatrist Abram Hoffer pioneered megavitamin research and treatment back in the early 1950s. Half a century later, his work still has been largely ignored by the medical profession. Dr. Hoffer has treated a whole lot of ADHD kids with vitamins.

It works.

I know a ten-year-old boy who was having considerable school and behavior problems. Interestingly enough, the child was already on physician-prescribed doses of niacin, but the total daily dose was only 150 mg. Not a bad beginning, since the RDA for kids is less than 20 mg per day. But it wasn't enough to be effective, and the boy was slated for the Ritalin-for-lunch bunch. Dr. Hoffer suggested giving him 500 mg niacinamide three times a day (1,500 mg total). That's a lot, but niacinamide is a comfortable, flush-free form of vitamin B_3. So Mom tried it. It helped greatly.

Then, she upped the dose to 3,000 mg per day. What a difference! The boy slept better, and his nightmares went away. He had fewer emotional meltdowns during the day and was less argumentative, less hyper, and less aggressive. He was warmer and more loving with his parents and more tolerant of changes in his routine. Basically, he reverted to the normal, happy-kid behavior that you just cannot buy in a Ritalin bottle.

People often ask, "If this treatment is so good, how come my doctor doesn't know about it? How come it is not on the news?" The answer may have more to do with medical politics than with medical science. Dr. Hoffer writes this about Attention Deficit Hyperactivity Disorder: "The DSM system [the standard of the American Psychiatric Association] has little or no relevance to diagnosis. It has no relevance to treatment, either, because no matter which terms are used to classify these children, they are all recommended for treatment with drug therapy" combined, sometimes, with other non-megavitamin approaches. "If the entire diagnostic scheme were scrapped today, it would make almost no difference to the way these children were treated, or to the outcome of treatment. Nor would their patients feel any better or worse." Statements like these do not exactly endear one to the medical community.

As if such statements are not enough, Dr. Hoffer has devoted an entire book (*Dr. Hoffer's ABC of Natural Nutrition for Children,* Quarry Press, 1999) to setting out genuine nutritional alternatives to drug therapy for ADHD children. He provides vitamin dosage details, food tables, and over 150 references. In addition, 120 case histories are included, along with a "bad foods" list, numerous research summaries, precise recommendations for optimum diet, comparisons of drugs and vitamins, a discussion of allergies and food additives, behavioral self-tests, and, most important, a wealth of professional experience.

Criticisms and even lawsuits over the hazards of tranquilizers, Ritalin, and behavior-modifying pharmaceuticals are on the rise, but neither court nor controversy can cure your child. "Battered parents" (Hoffer's term) need to know what to do, and *now.* Saying no to drugs also requires saying "yes" to something else. That something else is nutrition, properly employed.

For those who say there is insufficient scientific evidence to support megavitamin therapy for children's behavior disorders, I say they haven't been looking hard enough. Hoffer and his colleagues conducted the first double-blind controlled vitamin trials in psychiatric history in 1952. He was among the first to employ vitamin C as an antioxidant, to use the B vitamins against heart disease, and to employ niacin to treat behavioral disorders.

In light of this, organized medicine's "try everything but megavitamins" philosophy remains a puzzler, but it isn't the bottom line. This, however, is: The simple way to determine whether vitamins will help your child is to try them. A good place to start is with "Saul's Super Remedy" at the beginning of Part Two.

What is important is the weight of evidence that impelled me to take the steps
I did. My personal actions may not have justified the evidence,
but I think the evidence justified my actions.

ROGER J. WILLIAMS, PH.D., *NUTRITION AGAINST DISEASE*

She was a very nice lady, the wife of a surgeon, and an incurable alcoholic. Betty, age fifty-six, had been in and out of every rehab facility you can name. The famous ones, the expensive ones: all the king's horses and all the king's men couldn't seem to stop her from drinking again.

But its no joke, not at all. One in three American adults does not drink any alcoholic beverages. One third drinks very moderately and responsibly. And one third of all American adults drinks too much. Ten percent of our population can be classified as very heavy drinkers, putting down half of all alcohol consumed in the nation.

So Betty is not alone. But it seemed strange at first as she sat there in front of me, gracious and poised, telling me of her misery. Most of my experience with alcoholics came from volunteering at an urban soup kitchen. There, the winos fit the stereotype much better: disheveled men slurping from bottles of blackberry brandy in filthy paper bags. Truth is, you will not recognize most alcoholics. Most manage, somehow, to cope. This is easiest if they have money and free time, which means that many have gray hair. Believe it or not, 70 percent of elderly hospitalizations in 1991 were for alcohol-related problems.

"Is there anything you can do for me?" Betty asked.

Yeah, right, I thought to myself. Nobody had had any lasting luck getting this lady off the sauce. And you think you're gonna do it, fella? Pull the other leg.

Then the little cartoon angel whispered in my other ear. Roger J. Williams!

"There is a proven nutritional treatment for alcoholism," I said. "Roger Williams, a chemistry professor at the University of Texas and former president of the American Chemical Society, has written extensively on the subject. His work dates as far back as the 1950s, but is still as practical as if written yesterday."

"What does he recommend?" Betty asked.

"Megadoses of vitamins and an amino acid called L-glutamine. You might want to write this down. Thousands of milligrams of vitamin C a day, in divided doses; all the B vitamins, especially thiamine, in a B-complex supplement, five times a day; and about three grams of L-glutamine. This, plus a general good diet, with an avoidance of sugar, is essentially it. Can you do it?"

Betty smiled. "The real question is, will I do it, isn't it?"

17

"Yes," I said. "You've tried everything else."

Some weeks later I got an encouraging phone call from Betty. "Things are going great," she said. "Haven't had a drink since the day I saw you."

"Terrific!" But will she keep it going? I wondered. "Remember that the supplements won't do any good in the bottle. You've got to stay with this permanently, you know."

Months passed. A Christmas card from Betty: she was still clean and sober, she wrote. Next year, another Christmas card told of her continued success. "I'm going back to school," she wrote. Nice! "I've been able to have a drink or two now and again," Betty added, and the bottom fell right out of my happy mood. "But I stop when I choose, and do not want any more than that. I'm still taking all the vitamins. Thank you again!"

Once more, my understanding of alcoholism was overturned. Professional dogma tells us that "once an alcoholic, always an alcoholic." I've taught alcohol and substance abuse classes at the college level as part of a certified alcohol counselor training program. I know the drill, and Betty's experience did not fit well. She should not drink at all! Never!

Yet here she was, able to have a drink just like a normal person. She could choose to have a drink, and then stop. No compulsion, no addiction. Betty wasn't just coping better; she wasn't just recovering. Betty was cured.

Dr. Williams is responsible for the key nutritional concept, ignored by the medical and dietetic professions, that different people need differing amounts of nutrients. One size never fits all; anyone who has ever bought underwear will tell you this. Even people the same size and age will require differing amounts of nutrients, due to lifestyle and genetic factors. An alcoholic, for example, needs vastly more of certain vitamins than a non-drinker. There is a reason for this.

Beverage alcohol is ethanol, C_2H_5OH. It is a simple carbohydrate, much like sugar, supplying lots of energy and no other nutrients. Thiamine (vitamin B_1) is needed for carbohydrate metabolism. Extra carbs, including extra alcohol, require extra thiamine. Because alcohol is filling, it displaces more nourishing foods in the diet, causing malnutrition and specifically causing thiamine deficiency.

So the heavy drinker is much less likely to get even the usual dietary amount of thiamine, at a time when she needs much more. Add to this the fact that alcohol destroys the liver and brain gradually, but profoundly. This damage increases the need for nutrients to repair the body at a time when the drinker is eating fewer and fewer good foods. Still worse, alcohol causes poor absorption and utilization of what few B vitamins are coming in. Alcohol can literally destroy folic acid.

A deficiency of thiamine, just thiamine, produces the following symptoms, according to the respected textbook *Nutrition and Diet Therapy:*

Gastrointestinal: anorexia, indigestion, severe constipation, gastric atony, and insufficient stomach-acid secretion. (All of these result mostly from a lack of energy to the GI tract cells; no thiamine, no energy, no function.)

Cardiovascular: dilation of peripheral blood vessels (edema), weakened heart muscle, and heart failure.

Neurological: diminished reflex response, reduced alertness, fatigue, apathy. Continued deficiency produces damage or degeneration to myelin sheaths (fatty nerve-cell insulation material).

If you see an obvious tie-in to multiple sclerosis, you're right. A lack of thiamine causes increased nerve irritation, pain, prickly sensations, deadening sensations, and, if unchecked, paralysis. Thiamine-deficiency nerve damage can result in the DTs and hallucinations.

All this, mind you, from a deficiency of just one vitamin.

The U.S. thiamine RDA of a milligram or two is not remotely enough. A very strong case can be made for 25 to 65 mg per day even for nonalcoholics. The heavy drinker's poor diet, plus ensuing alcohol damage, plus increased thiamine need proportional to carbohydrate intake points to an optimum B_1 intake of several hundred milligrams per day.

One study of about two thousand households for a full year showed that more than 65 percent of adults got less than the RDA of thiamine. This means that half to two-thirds of Americans probably are thiamine-deficient even if they do not drink at all. Thiamine is found in almost all natural foods, but in tiny amounts. Precious few sober Americans, let alone alcoholics, eat large quantities of the whole grains and legumes (peas, beans, and lentils) that are modest food sources of thiamine.

Therefore, vitamin B_1 supplements are essential. To get maximum results, additional nutrients must also be provided in abundance through supplementation.

Which ones, specifically?

1. Vitamin C in great quantity (on the order of 10,000 to 20,000 mg per day and more). High doses of vitamin C chemically neutralize the toxic byproducts of alcohol metabolism. Vitamin C also increases the liver's ability to reverse the fatty buildup so common in alcoholics.

2. B complex, consisting of 50 mg of each of the major B vitamins, six times daily. The B-complex vitamins work best in concert with each other.

3. L-glutamine, 2,000 to 3,000 mg per day. This amino acid helps decrease physiological cravings for alcohol.

4. Lecithin, 2 to 4 tablespoons daily. This provides inositol and choline, which are related to the B complex. Lecithin also helps mobilize fats out of the liver.

5. Chromium, at least 200 to perhaps 400 mcg chromium polynicotinate daily. Chromium greatly improves carbohydrate metabolism and helps control blood sugar levels. Many, if not most, alcoholics are hypoglycemic.

6. A good high-potency multivitamin, multimineral supplement as well, containing magnesium (400 mg) and the antioxidants carotene and vitamin E (d-alpha-tocopherol).

19

Dr. Ruth Harrell elegantly confirmed Dr. Williams's theory when she gave huge doses of vitamins, especially B complex, to severely mentally handicapped children. She obtained extraordinary improvement in learning and IQ in a matter of months, including spectacular advances in Down's syndrome children. This work was done in 1981 and published in the *Proceedings of the National Academy of Sciences.*

Why, then, does the medical establishment keep Dr. Williams's knowledge filed away, out of sight? The answer is classic: follow the money.

In America, there is a vested interest in disease. There is no profit in prevention. You make a whole lot more money treating alcoholism than you do not having alcoholism. It is the very "social cost" of this, and other diseases, that makes them profitable. It is a tough concept, but think about it: There is a shortage of special education teachers! America's courts and prisons are backlogged and overcrowded! Nursing homes have waiting lists! There are waiting lists for organ transplants! Medical costs are through the roof! What can we conclude? Simple: Business is good! In a PBS news program entitled *Affluenza,* the point is made that every time a person is diagnosed with cancer, the nation's Gross Domestic Product goes up.

So what are we to do, at least those of us who want results? The first rule of fishing is to put your hook in the water, for that is where the fish are. Try Roger Williams's protocol, and see what I saw with Betty.

When someone becomes unconscious from ethanol, they may have had just enough to pass out, or they may have had just enough to die. One cannot afford to take a chance and see if they sleep it off, or never wake. To stop such emergencies from occurring, we also cannot afford to ignore vitamin therapy.

*I don't know if the world is full of smart men bluffing
or imbeciles who mean it.*

ATTRIBUTED TO MORRIE BRICKMAN

Most allergies are a lot of bunk. They usually disappear while you wait if you use the safest, cheapest, and most effective antihistamine-antitoxin in existence: vitamin C. I know, you don't believe me. How could a simple vitamin replace a medical specialty? Yet it's true. You could start a drive-in allergy clinic with only one prescription: "Take C. Forty dollars, please. Do you want fries with that?"

Wisdom is inherent in simplicity and safety. Hippocrates, the father of so-called medicine, said, "Of several remedies, the physician should choose the least sensational." That is genius, and it is practical advice good for modern man. Vitamin C therapy is safe, simple, and effective.

So you question this naive approach? Naturally, since we've all been taught that anything safe and simple cannot possibly be medically effective. So I give you the case of my friend Tim.

Tim brought in his wife and family to talk about scarlet fever. They'd had a touch of it in their family—and a touch is enough of that. We discussed vitamin C's role as an antipyretic (fever-reducer) and value as an antibiotic. They were keen to focus on this. In passing, Tim also mentioned some unspecified allergy problems. I briefly mentioned that vitamin C had great usefulness there as well.

Tim called me a few weeks later. "Good resolution with the fever," he said. "We gave all the kids grams of vitamin C and only one of them had scarlet fever symptoms. That was Jeffrey, and he got over it much faster than the doctor expected him to."

"That's really good, Tim," I said.

"There's more to tell," he responded. "I was stung by a bee last week."

"And?"

"And I'm allergic to bee stings."

Ulp. He hadn't previously told me that.

"I have medicine and an inhaler," Tim continued. "The whole kit and kaboodle. When I was stung, I took 25,000 mg of vitamin C in the first hour. By the end of the day, I'd taken 100,000 mg. No symptoms at all. Not even any swelling. You had to look hard to find where the sting was."

"But you used your medicine, right?"

"No!" Tim said. "That's the amazing thing. Normally I would have had to, or I would probably die. But this time, all I did was the C. Talk about an antitoxin-antihistamine! That stuff really works."

I was unnerved at the high stakes Tim had played for, but impressed with his findings.

Allergy, like most disease names, tells you little about cause and nothing about cure. Robert F. Cathcart, M.D., looks at allergy (and many other conditions, as well) simply in terms of how much vitamin C it takes to cure it. He has much experience as a clinician and has published numerous papers on the topic.

And he is correct.

A twenty-year-old woman once saw me about her allergies to horses and hay. Since she loved to ride, and her parents kept several horses in their barn, this was a big problem. The young lady was not readily going to change her eating habits, but was willing to take a lot of vitamin C. It was effective, as she tells it:

"Whenever I was taking 20,000 mg of vitamin C a day, I had no allergies at all. The only time I got them back was when I drank beer. So I either avoided beer, or if I drank, I took an extra 10,000 mg of C. I never had problems with horses or hay again."

I once had a client who was allergic to everything, literally. She'd tested out positive as allergic to seventy-two different substances. I'd never heard of that severe a condition before, and neither had her allergist. He said that she could take a "megadose" of perhaps 1,000 mg a day. It was not doing anything. I suggested she take vitamin C to bowel tolerance, and hold the C level just below the amount that caused loose stools. This turned out to be nearly 40,000 mg a day. She took all the C she could hold. That was the end of her seventy-two allergies.

And I've seen more of the same with children and teenagers, friends and neighbors, all ages and stages. Take enough C to be symptom free, whatever the amount might be . . . but stay a few thousand milligrams under the amount that causes diarrhea. That's about your only concern, because the safety of vitamin C therapy is unassailable. Dr. Frederick Robert Klenner writes, "Vitamin C is the safest substance available to the physician."

I've got another story for you. Back in the 1970s, Dr. Benjamin Feingold, an allergist, noticed that some children seemed to be noticeably sensitive to artificial colors and other food additives. He worked primarily with hyperactive kids, had their parents clean up their diets and go chemical-free, and the hyperactive behavior stopped. From this came a classic book, *Why Your Child Is Hyperactive.*

Feingold was an M.D., credentialed in every way and then some. Feingold's diet was so effective that Feingold Associations—grassroots groups of parents—sprung up across the nation. Basically, all they did was keep painted foods out of their children's stomachs.

The food industry's response was predictable. Study after study has been bankrolled to show that food additives—and sugar, for that matter—have no negative effect on children's behavior. Yeah, right! Been to a kid's birthday party lately? Ever taught school during the week following Halloween? Ever tried to nap a toddler full of M&M's? Most important, did you ever read Feingold's book? This man knows what he is talking about and got good results. As long as we let kids eat chemically dyed foods and drinks, we might just as well give them a can of Sherwin-Williams housepaint and a spoon.

The worst that can be said about the Feingold approach is that it doesn't work for all children. Somewhere around half of all kids will improve on his program. Maybe it is no more than a placebo effect. But it is still worth a try because there is no harm to it. Doctors give chemotherapy with a success rate of under 30 percent, and chemo has serious side effects. What is the down side of not feeding kids food paint? How can it possibly hurt to try avoidance of unneeded chemicals?

What really rankles me is that allergists have made a subculture out of avoiding various molds, pollens, hairs, foods—all substances to which we have had millions of years of evolutionary exposure. Allergists will be quick to tell you that your child is allergic—but not, of course, to an industrial synthetic chemical dye. For it would somehow seem to them that only substances found in nature can produce an authentic allergy. Factory foods and artificial colors bearing molecular names a yard long cannot *possibly* cause hyperactivity.

And remember, everyone: giving sugar to a hyper child is perfectly okay! Logic like that does not even pass the straight-faced test.

Imagine what would actually happen if everyone were healthy. If each person ate right and took vitamins. If doctors and hospitals and pharmaceuticals, all of which prosper from sickness, were not needed. In America, there is a vested interest in disease. There is no profit in prevention.

The United States Recommended Dietary Allowances (or Reference Intakes, or whatever other claptrap they offer you) are forms of nutritional communism. According to them, the government-set levels are ample for all, and that's the end of it. A socialist state might say that you only need a subsistence income, say a few thousand dollars above the federal poverty level. Would your needs be met with ten thousand dollars a year? Would you be best off that way? Or would you like the right to try to get more? Does the government have either the knowledge, or the right, to decide either your financial needs or your nutritional needs?

When it comes to RDAs, one size fits nobody. Let's temporarily assume that orthodox dietitians are correct when they tell us that vitamin supplements can cure nothing but vitamin deficiency diseases. If this is true, then any symptom cured by supplements indicates a deficiency. If zinc speeds recovery from the common cold (and many studies confirm this), then people with colds are zinc-deficient. If lots of vitamin C shortens the intensity and duration of the common cold (and dozens of scientific studies prove this), then people with colds are vitamin C deficient as well. The RDAs and pitiful American intakes are therefore below the deficiency levels.

LAW: The quantity of a nutritional supplement that cures an illness indicates the patient's degree of deficiency. It is therefore not a megadose of the vitamin, but rather a megadeficiency of the nutrient, that we are dealing with.

23

Allergies evidently constitute one such megadeficiency.

You must use vitamins correctly to get the job done. Large amounts work; small amounts don't. The dose depends on the patient. Dr. Klenner said, "If you want results, use adequate ascorbic acid. Don't send a boy to do a man's job." If I were to die tomorrow, I'd want you to remember that I told you this today: "Take enough C to be symptom-free, whatever that amount might be." (It even rhymes, making your job easier.)

I raised my kids all the way into college without either of them ever having a single dose of an antibiotic. Why? Because we used vitamins instead, that's why. And this especially meant lots of vitamin C. Vitamin C very effectively treated their influenzas and mononucleosis; it promptly stopped their coughs and bronchitis; it lowered their fevers and cured their sore throats. I repeat: they never once had an antibiotic. Because of the C, they never once needed an antibiotic.

Vitamin C is but one of many vitamins, vitamins are but one part of nutrition, and nutrition is but one aspect of health. But look at what just one vitamin can do. *At saturation (bowel tolerance) levels, vitamin C replaces antibiotics, antihistamines, antipyretics, antitoxics, and antiviral drugs.* This is one of the most inflammatory statements in medicine.

An English friend of mine told me that he'd hardly even heard of allergies until he came to the United States. "Allergies were quite rare in Britain," he said. "In America it seems everyone has them, children especially." He's right. If you asked grandma, she might say the whole allergy business is ridiculous. I agree with grandma. I think there is only one genuine allergy, and that involves the fatal result of transfusing the wrong type of blood into a person. Anything else is simple by comparison, and deserving of nutritional therapy.

What we now label "allergies" could just as easily be called "undernutrition" and I think should be. The majority of Americans eat lousy diets; nine out of ten of us do not meet even the already low RDA levels for fruit and vegetable vitamins. Insufficient vitamin C results in exaggerated sensitivity to even average levels of irritants, toxins, chemicals, pollution, and microorganisms. Deficiencies of vitamins A, B complex, and E frequently manifest as skin problems or hypersensitivity to foods, stress, or germs. Millions of vitamin-deficient but overstuffed people are literally waiting to be allergic to something. Food that fills and fattens but doesn't fortify the body is like trying to build a wall with bricks but no mortar: it will hold up only until you lean upon it.

If your son got sweaty palms or hives every time he telephoned a girl to ask her for a date, would you conclude that he's allergic to women and send him to a monastery? Of course not. You'd find out why he got so nervous and strengthen him, encourage him, and most of all allow him to get over it. So why not do the same for your body?

An allergy is a symptom, and symptoms tell us that our body is not quite right. Naturopaths tell us that if our body is not quite right, we should take a good look at the way we take care of it. Check your diet first, not for the presence of allergens but for an absence of nutrients. You can start with a saturation test with vitamin C, as mentioned above.

Other questions to ask yourself: Are you avoiding chemical preservatives and other unnecessary food additives? Avoiding drugs, nonprescription and otherwise? Are you getting enough rest? Do you need a cleansing fast? These questions should replace battery after battery of allergy tests.

In my opinion, the way to be healthy is deceptively simple:

1. Stop eating meat, sugar, and artificially colored junk food, or at least reduce intake of these substances as much as possible.

2. Instead, eat whole grains, fruits, beans, sprouts, lightly cooked or raw vegetables, and regularly take vitamin food supplements (especially vitamin C).

3. Clean out body wastes by occasional juice fasts and an everyday natural diet that is high in fiber and free of artificially colored or preserved foods.

This is more than folk medicine. It is a real remedy for all folks.

But don't just take my word for it. A whole host of reputable doctors have championed the virtues of C. Here are some of the best: *How to Live Longer and Feel Better,* by Linus Pauling; *Vitamin C, Infectious Diseases, and Toxins: Curing the Incurable,* by Thomas E. Levy; *Clinical Guide to the Use of Vitamin C,* edited by Lendon Smith; *The Vitamin C Connection,* by Emanuel Cheraskin; *A Physician's Handbook on Orthomolecular Medicine,* edited by Roger Williams; and *Orthomolecular Psychiatry,* by David Hawkins and Linus Pauling. Do not be dismayed by these highfalutin titles. "Orthomolecular" is just another term for megavitamin.

Can you make your allergies disappear forever? To find out, follow the plan I lay out in "Saul's Super Remedy" in Part Two. It just may change your life.

F act: More than half the nursing-home beds in the United States are occupied by Alzheimer's patients. Fact: Alzheimer's disease is the number-four killer of Americans, causing over 100,000 deaths each year. I believe that many of these deaths are unnecessary; aggressive use of therapeutic nutrition could substantially reduce the incidence and severity of Alzheimer's disease. Let's take a look on a vitamin-by-vitamin basis.

Vitamin B_{12}

B_{12} deficiency may be mistaken for, or perhaps cause, Alzheimer's disease. Note how closely these symptoms of B_{12} deficiency mirror those of Alzheimer's: ataxia, fatigue, slowness of thought, apathy, emaciation, degeneration of the spinal cord, dizziness, moodiness, confusion, agitation, delusions, hallucinations, and psychosis. B_{12} deficiency is easy to come by in the elderly: poor diet; poor intestinal absorption (due to less intrinsic factor being secreted by the aging stomach, and possibly due to calcium deficiency); digestive tract surgery; pharmaceutical interference, notably from Dilantin (phenytoin); and stress all decrease B_{12}. It is necessary to measure the cerebrospinal fluid, not the blood, to get accurate B_{12} readings.

Even marginal B_{12} deficiency over an extended time produces an increased risk of Alzheimer's disease. Many popular dieting plans are B_{12} deficient, including the Pritikin, Scarsdale, and Beverly Hills diets. The elderly are often "dieting" without intending to, simply because their normal appetite and taste functions are reduced. Emotional factors such as isolation, grief, and depression also contribute to inadequate food intake, and therefore low B_{12} intake. To make matters worse, B_{12} deficiency itself causes further loss of appetite.

Injection or intranasal administration of B_{12} is the recommended method of supplementation because oral absorption is poor. There is no known toxicity for vitamin B_{12}. A minimum daily therapeutic dose is probably 100 mcg daily, and closer to 1,000 mcg may be more effective. 1,000 mcg sounds like a lot, but it is actually the same as 1 mg, which is about one thousandth of a quarter-teaspoon.

Choline

Alzheimer's patients have a deficiency of the neurotransmitter acetylcholine because they are deficient in the enzyme, choline acetyltransferase, needed to make it. But there is a way around this: increasing dietary choline raises blood and brain levels of acetylcholine. Choline is readily available in cheap, nonprescription lecithin. A large quantity of choline (from lecithin) is necessary for clinical results. Lecithin is nontoxic. Start with at least a heaping tablespoon daily, working up to a goal of three or four tablespoons each day.

Vitamin C, Tyrosine, and Other Vitamins

Increasing the body's level of the neurotransmitter norepinephrine may also help Alzheimer's patients. Norepinephrine is made from the amino acid tyrosine, which is made from phenylalanine. We get plenty of phenylalanine from protein in our diets if we eat protein foods, but the conversion to tyrosine and ultimately norepinephrine may not take place if there is a deficiency of another coenzyme: vitamin C, which is necessary for norepinephrine production. Vitamin C may therefore be of special value in the treatment of Alzheimer's.

Antioxidant vitamins, such as vitamin E and carotene, may slow down or prevent Alzheimer's. Alzheimer's patients have abnormally low levels of these nutrients in their bodies. This could simply be because they don't eat well, or because the disease increases their nutrient need, or both. Between 400 and 600 IU of vitamin E is a reasonable daily starting dose, with a gradual "test increase" to higher levels. A glass or two of carrot juice each day will take care of the carotene.

Deficiencies of thiamine, riboflavin, vitamin C, and pyridoxine (B_6) are frequently seen in the elderly, even among individuals using supplements. This indicates that the RDA levels for these vitamins need to be raised. Folic acid and niacin, as well as other nutrients, may also play a major role in combating Alzheimer's.

Consider a five-times-a day dose of a high potency B-complex supplement, with at least 500 to 1,000 mg of vitamin C on the hour.

Aluminum Toxicity

Unintentional intake of aluminum, a known neurotoxin, may increase the risk of Alzheimer's as well. Aluminum cookware, aluminum foil, antacids, douches, buffered aspirin, and even antiperspirant deodorants may contribute to the problem. A single aluminum coffeepot was shown to have invisibly added more than 1,600 mcg aluminum per liter of water. This is *thirty-two times* the World Health Organization's set goal of 50 mcg per liter. Aluminum is known to build up in the body tissues of people with Alzheimer's disease, Parkinson's disease, and amyotrophic lateral sclerosis. Aluminum is also a component of so-called "silver" amalgam dental fillings. Composite (white) fillings do not contain aluminum (or mercury, for that matter). Most baking powder contains aluminum. Rumford brand baking powder does not, however. Neither does baking soda, which is a different substance entirely.

Artificial kidney dialysis has been known to produce "dialysis dementia," a state of confusion and disorientation caused by excess aluminum in the blood stream. Animals injected with aluminum compounds will also develop nervous system disorders. Conversely, Alzheimer's disease can be treated with metal bonding (chelating) agents, such as desferrioxamine, which remove aluminum from the bloodstream. In appropriately high doses, vitamin C is also an effective (and nonprescription) chelating agent.

Calcium and magnesium significantly slow down aluminum absorption, and that's good. Supplementation with 800 mg of calcium and 400 mg of magnesium every day may be therapeutic for Alzheimer's patients. The citrate forms of these minerals are well absorbed and relatively inexpensive.

Lead Toxicity

An April 2000 presentation to the American Academy of Neurology showed that "people who have held jobs with high levels of lead exposure have a 3.4 times greater likelihood of developing Alzheimer's disease." Lead has adverse effects on brain development and function, even at very low levels of exposure. Lead, unfortunately, permeates our environment because of decades of adding it to gasoline. The good news is that very high doses of vitamin C are known to help the body rapidly excrete lead.

Recommended Reading

Alzheimer's disease and neurotransmitters. *Let's Live* (May 1983): 18.

Balch JF and Balch PA. *Prescription for Nutritional Healing.* Garden City Park, NY: Avery Publishing, 1990, 87–90.

Carper J. Your food pharmacy. [syndicated column] (1 November 1995).

Dommisse J. Organic mania induced by phenytoin. *Can J Psychiatry* 35 (June 1990).

Dommisse J. Subtle vitamin B_{12} deficiency and psychiatry: a largely unnoticed but devastating relationship? *Med Hypotheses* 34 (1991): 131–140.

Dooley E. Linking lead to Alzheimer's disease. *Environmental Health Perspectives* 108 (October 2000).

Fisher and Lachance. Nutrition evaluation of published weight reducing diets. *J Amer Dietetic Assn* 85 (1985): 450–54.

Garrison RH and Somer E. *The Nutrition Desk Reference.* New Canaan, CT: Keats Publishing, 1990, 78–79, 106, 210–211.

Goldberg D. *Newsletter* 33 (September 1985).

Jackson JA, Riordan HD, and Poling CM. Aluminum from a coffee pot. *Lancet* 8641 (8 April 1989): 781–782.

Kushnir SL, Ratner JT, and Gregoire PA. Multiple nutrients in the treatment of Alzheimer's disease. *Amer Geriatrics Soc J* 35 (May 1987): 476–477.

Little, et al. A double-blind, placebo controlled trial of high dose lecithin in Alzheimer's disease. *J Neurology, Neurosurgery and Psychiatry* 48 (1985): 736–742.

Martyn CN, et al. Geographical relation between Alzheimer's disease and aluminum in drinking water. *Lancet* 8629 (14 Jan 1989): 59–62.

McLachlan DR, Kruck TP, and Lukiw WJ. Would decreased aluminum ingestion reduce the incidence of Alzheimer's disease? *Can Med Assn J* (1 Oct 1991).

Murray F. A B$_{12}$ deficiency may cause mental problems. *Better Nutrition for Today's Living* (July 1991): 10–11.

Weiner MA. Aluminum and dietary factors in Alzheimer's disease. *J Orthomolecular Med* 5 (1990): 74–78.

Williams SR. *Nutrition and Diet Therapy,* 6th ed., St. Louis: Mosby, 1989, 250.

It was a bit odd to have a conversation with my sixty-seven-year-old father about his sex life.

"I'm on this medicine, Andrew," he said. "It's for angina. My doctor sent me to a heart specialist, and they both agreed I have to take it. The problem is that it causes impotence." I let that image sink in as he continued. "Are there any of your natural remedies that can replace the angina medicine?"

Now, it was an unusual event for my dad to ask my view about anything. One of his mottoes is, "If I want your opinion, I'll give it to you." So I was duly impressed with the gravity of the situation.

"Vitamin E, Pa, " I said. "High doses of vitamin E have been used to treat angina since the early fifties. Wilfrid and Evan Shute, who were brothers and cardiologists, gave patients somewhere between 1,600 and 2,000 international units of vitamin E daily and it eliminated angina symptoms in hundreds and hundreds of documented cases."

I fully expected him to ridicule the idea, and I was surprised and not a little gratified when he thoughtfully nodded his head. "Okay," he said, and we eagerly moved on to another topic.

My dad started at about 400 IU a day, gradually working up to 1,600 IU over a period of a few weeks. I've always maintained that the body likes gradual change. This goes for decreasing drugs as well as for increasing vitamins. Pa's general practitioner was an open-minded man, quite British and quite willing to offer my father a dosage-reduction schedule for his medication.

And that is all it took.

Pa called a couple of weeks later. "Is it all right to take this much vitamin E?" he asked.

"How much are you up to?"

"Uh, 1,200 a day."

"How do you feel?"

"Pretty fair," he said. "I'm practically off the medication now."

"Any symptoms?" I asked.

"No."

"Why don't you go to 1,600 with no drugs," I said.

The subject did not come up again for months. What can I say? This is how our family does things.

"So, Pa, how's that angina?" I asked one day.

"What angina?" he said.

"*Your* angina, Pa."

"I don't have angina."

"Well you did. Maybe a year ago."

"I never had any angina," he said.

"Two doctors said you did, Pa. They had you on medication, remember?"

"Oh, that. I haven't had any sign of that since I took the vitamin E."

"OK. Keep taking the E, Pa."

"I do. 1,600 every day."

And that was that. He never had angina symptoms again.

Usually the fur really flies when you bring up the Shute brothers' vitamin E treatment for cardiovascular disease. This has been a controversial area of medicine for sixty years. Most textbooks state that "E" is of no value here. Textbooks have said for years that vitamin E is a quack's cure in search of a disease. But there is considerable evidence that the texts are wrong and the Shutes were right.

Consider intermittent claudication, which is calf-muscle pain upon walking. Even conventional nutrition textbooks acknowledge scientific proof of this successful treatment with vitamin E. "This therapy helps reduce the arterial blockage," says Williams in *Nutrition and Diet Therapy,* a standard dietetics work. Is there something so special about the arteries between the knee and the ankle? What about "reducing the blockage" in other arteries? This is the whole idea of using Vitamin E for circulatory diseases.

Medical doctors Wilfrid and Evan Shute of London, Ontario, successfully treated well over 30,000 cardiovascular disease patients with up to 3,200 IU of vitamin E daily. They were rewarded for that achievement by being ostracized from their medical society. Here are the principles of the therapy:

1. Vitamin E has an oxygen-sparing effect on the heart, enabling the heart to do more work on less oxygen. The benefit for recovering heart-attack patients is considerable. 1,200–2,000 IU daily relieves angina very well.

2. Vitamin E moderately prolongs prothrombin clotting time, and has a limited Coumadin/warfarin effect, "thinning" the blood but, unlike the drugs, not doing so beyond normal limits. This is the reason behind the Shutes' using vitamin E for thrombophlebitis and related conditions. Their dose? About 1,000–2,000 IU daily.

3. Vitamin E dilates and promotes collateral circulation and benefits diabetes patients or anyone threatened with gangrene. Dose: tailored to patient; 800 IU daily or more.

4. Vitamin E strengthens and regulates heartbeat like digitalis (foxglove) and its derivatives at a dose adjusted to 800–3,000 IU daily.

5. Vitamin E reduces scarring when frequently applied topically to burns or sites of lacerations or surgical incisions along with a daily oral dose of 800 IU.

6. Vitamin E helps gradually break down clots at a maintained daily dose of 800–3,000 IU.

7. Vitamin E is vastly safer than drugs, as doses of up to 56,000 IU per day fail to harm adult humans. Gradual dosage increase is advised, and patients with congestive heart failure, rheumatic hearts, or high blood pressure need careful medical supervision.

So why hasn't vitamin E been more highly regarded in medicine? Ambiguous results from a rather small number of highly publicized, poorly controlled studies, that's why. The most common reason for irreproducibility of successful vitamin E cures is either a failure to use enough or a failure to use the natural d-alpha (as opposed to dl-alpha) form, or both. Such studies must be weighed against the Shutes' 30,000 cured patients and their four books: *Complete Updated Vitamin E Book, Health Preserver, Vitamin E for Ailing and Healthy Hearts,* and *Your Child and Vitamin E.*

In less healthy people, there are some valid cautions in giving large doses of vitamin E. Among hypertensive patients, sudden large vitamin E increases cause temporary increases in blood pressure. The solution is to increase the vitamin gradually, with proper monitoring (which hypertensive patients should have anyway). To avoid any possible risks of an asymmetric heart contraction, patients with rheumatic hearts or congestive heart failure need small doses (around 75 IU) and increases under medical supervision. It is best to inquire about all of these conditions when taking or submitting a patient history. For additional information, it is most worthwhile to contact the Shute Institute in London, Ontario, or to read any books by Wilfrid or Evan Shute.

Why supplement with vitamin E? Our need for vitamin E increases with advanced age, exposure to toxins (smoking, air pollution, chemical oxidants), pregnancy, and lactation. Even an increased consumption of polyunsaturated fats requires more vitamin E to protect the unsaturated fatty acids from free-radical attack. For most healthy adults, an optimum daily amount of vitamin E would probably be about 600 IU. It must certainly be higher than the RDA of only about 10 or 15 IU.

True, many foods contain vitamin E, including dairy products, eggs, meat, fish, whole-grain cereals and whole-grain breads, wheat germ, and leafy vegetables. However, only very small quantities of the vitamin are present in these foods. Americans do not get enough vitamin E in their diet, and it is impossible to get even 100 IU per day from the finest of diets. This is at least partly due to the widespread refining of flour since the start of the twentieth century. Heart disease has also been on a steep increase since 1900. Very likely there is a connection here.

The New England Journal of Medicine published two papers in the May 20, 1993, issue (vol. 328, pp. 1,444–1,456) that supported vitamin E megadoses, reporting an approximate 40 percent reduction in cardiovascular disease. Nearly 40,000 men and 87,000 women took part in the study. The more vitamin E they took, and the longer they took it, the less cardiovascular disease they experienced.

And the Shute brothers, those quacks, pointed it out first—sixty years ago. They said, "We didn't make vitamin E this versatile. God did. Ignore it at your peril."

And ignore it we have. The very same issue of *The New England Journal of Medicine* that carried the two favorable vitamin E studies included another piece on this amazing vitamin: an editorial, advising doctors not to use it. One can only wonder why.

Warning: keep this medicine out of the reach of everybody!
Use vitamin C instead!

LINUS PAULING, TWO-TIME RECIPIENT OF THE NOBEL PRIZE

Any physician who gives twelve courses of antibiotics to an infant is a real quack. I know more than one doctor who does.

Ray, a health professional himself, brought his eleven-month-old son Robbie to me. The child was very sick, and had been so for more than a week. No one, and I mean no one, in their family had had any sleep in a long time. They were up night after night with this child, who had a high fever, glazed watery eyes, tons of thick mucus, and labored breathing. The poor child could not sleep and did little else but cry. Day and night, night and day.

Robbie was under the care of a pediatrician who had been prescribing some very serious antibiotics all along. Antibiotics were clearly not working. This was all too apparent to Ray. "Twelve rounds of antibiotics for a baby under a year old, and all the doctor wants to do is give more?" he said. "That makes no sense at all."

"Ray, antibiotics are their knee-jerk answer to a lot of things. When the only tool you have is a hammer, you tend to see every problem as a nail."

"Well, we've thoroughly tried the medical route, and cooperated one hundred percent with the pediatrician. At this point, Robbie is worse, not better. We've got to do something ourselves, and we are going to. My wife is just as emphatic about that as I am." (She was home, taking care of the other children.)

I promptly acquainted Ray with the vitamin C quacks. He agreed to give Robbie as much vitamin C as he could hold without having loose bowels.

So now I have a new case history record to offer: 20,000 mg of vitamin C daily for a twenty-pound baby of eleven months of age. That's how much it took to cure Ray's baby of severe congestion, fever, and listlessness. That is 1,000 mg of vitamin C per pound per day; nearly twice what Dr. Frederick Robert Klenner customarily ordered for patients. And even at that huge amount, the baby never had diarrhea!

You have to marvel at where it all went. More marvelous is how quickly it worked.

"Robbie was noticeably improved in under twelve hours, and slept through the first night," Ray told me two days later. "He was completely well in forty-eight hours. Symptom-free. Completely well!"

Even without considering the harmful side effects of massive antibiotic therapy, we can look at the futility of all those repeated doses. Antibiotics are either going to work with the first or second round, or they are not going to work at all, period. There is no point in emptying twelve fire extinguishers filled with water on an electrical fire. More of the wrong thing is just more wrong. And in a baby, just plain stupid.

The vitamin C quacks (Linus Pauling, Frederick Klenner, Emanuel Cheraskin, William J. McCormick, Irwin Stone, Thomas E. Levy, Robert F. Cathcart III, and, ah, me) will tell you that you have a genuine option: use vitamin C as your first choice antibiotic. Taking enough C results in the three Cs: patient comfort, low cost, and parental control.

Because of the medical profession's customarily paternalistic, condescending attitude toward self-care, your choosing vitamin C therapy will be denounced as irresponsible. It takes some real strength for a parent to stand firm and say, "This is what I am going to do: I am going to follow the Klenner/Cathcart vitamin C protocol." Knowing that all you risk is derision from the medical community makes it a little easier.

When I was a kid, everybody got miracle drugs. From sulfa to Physohex, we followed the crowd from waiting room to prescription counter. Our parents gave us "safe" children's aspirin. Oops, not so safe for high fevers, it was discovered. So then it was children's Tylenol (acetaminophen) for everybody. Hmm . . . turns out there's some liver and kidney side effects with that, too. All drugs carry side effects; you just choose your poison carefully. Vitamins are vastly safer.

LAW: The number-one side effect of vitamins is failure to take enough of them.

If you do choose to employ antibiotic drugs, bear in mind that they interfere with normal digestion by killing off beneficial colon bacteria. These are the very bacteria that make vitamin K and the B vitamins cobalamin and biotin, and that help us digest many plant and dairy foods, strengthen the immune system, and repress the overgrowth of pathogenic microorganisms. After antibiotic therapy, all persons should take yogurt and an acidophilus supplement for a month or two to help restore a normal, healthy bowel environment. I have found shamefully few doctors who tell this to their patients.

And this is not just about antibiotics. In the 1980 *Physicians' Desk Reference,* Prednisone didn't even have the diamond symbol of a frequently prescribed drug next to its listing. Now it is used almost indiscriminately. For instance, I know a sixteen-year-old girl who had a lousy diet, innumerable colds, and chronic bronchitis. After bucketfuls of antibiotics, the HMO doctors put her on Prednisone. Prednisone is a drug of desperation. When they pull out the corticosteroids, they don't know what else to do. Prednisone can cause the following nutritional problems, among others: sodium and fluid retention, potassium loss, osteoporosis, carbohydrate intolerance and increased insulin requirement, and a variety of gastrointestinal complications. Why subject a teenage kid to this?

On the other hand, I have in my possession two *United States Pharmacopoeia* statements on vitamin C for injection asserting that "there are no contraindications for the use of ascorbic acid (vitamin C)." Not to mention the fact that it works. Intelligently employing vitamins can eliminate many dangerous side effects that come from over-reliance on over-the-counter and prescription drugs.

This goes for viruses, too. Right now there are a whole lot of researchers searching for a good antiviral drug. They already have one. The pharmaceutical industry's mercenary scientists and their medical doctor clones will, in fact, try everything but mega-doses of vitamin C. I think of them as birds that are willing to land on any branch except one. Too bad, because that one branch is the best on the tree.

To treat infections with vitamin C, follow the guidelines listed in the chapter "Vitamin C Megadose Therapy."

If Dracula were an old woman, he would have sounded a lot like Mrs. Kelremor. Just shy of eighty, this Central European immigrant had been a housekeeper for decades. Overweight, worn out, and weighted down with cares, she came to see me primarily because of osteoarthritis.

It was the 1980s: disco was still considered music, and arthritis was still said to have no nutritional connection or cure. For centuries, quacks have known otherwise. Today, more and more, the medical profession is finally catching on. But Mrs. Kelremor couldn't wait for them. She said to me, in her thick Transylvanian accent, "I can't vork. I om avake all night. I om in pain all oof da time."

I vill now drop the accent; you get the picture.

Mrs. Kelremor bowed her gray-haired head as she continued speaking. "Look at my hands. I can't close them anymore. Look at my knees, all swollen. I am sore all over." As if that were not enough, she showed me an assortment of lumps on her arms and legs. Her doctor had told her they were benign. They certainly were not pleasant to behold. "What can I do?" she said. "My husband does not work. I have to work. I have to clean."

I suggested a real dietary overhaul, beginning with vegetable-juice fasting. There is a fine line between irresponsible promises and stimulating encouragement. I attempted to straddle that line by telling her that she had little to risk with vegetables.

She looked up, for the first time during the interview, and slowly said, "I will try anything."

Anything? Even living on raw vegetable juices eight days in a row, followed by very light eating for three days and a raw-food diet for the next ten? Repeatedly? For weeks and weeks?

"Yes," she said. "Anything."

The drop-out rate in such a program is high. That is probably the only true drawback of an otherwise venerable, simple, and safe program. To many, juice fasting conjures up images of starvation, electrolyte imbalance, malnutrition, and exhaustion. All false, and for very elementary reasons.

First, vegetables are especially nourishing foods, and a variety of vegetables guarantees more than adequate nutrition. The fact that they are juiced does not change that. Second, you cannot hurt yourself with produce. There is no down side to a vegetable diet, particularly when accompanied with a couple of good multivitamin pills each day. Eventually you'll want to reintroduce some legumes, sprouts, and nuts to your diet, for their protein, but that is after you've cleansed yourself through juicing.

So adequate nutrition—far more than adequate nutrition, really—can be maintained for weeks at a time on veggies alone. "But why juice? Why not just eat the vegetables?" Because you won't, that's why. Juicing guarantees quantity. If you juice, you simply will consume more vegetables. It is quicker and easier to down the juice than to sit and graze a table's worth of produce, so you will consume more. Additionally, the absorption of juiced vegetables is excellent, far superior to what you can get after just using your choppers to chew. Not being ruminants, like cows or giraffes, we get only one chance to masticate our food. A juicer does the job vastly better.

So that's it, then. A safe therapy that is too simple to work.

But it does. And the wretchedly bent-over Mrs. Kelremor was willing to try it.

Not without a fight, however. For weeks, I got her phone calls. "Can I have soup?"

Sure, if it will please you.

"Can I have some sausage?"

No.

"Can I cook some of the vegetables?"

Some vegetables have to be cooked, such as sweet potatoes and, moving away from a strict meaning of the word *vegetable*, beans and rice. If some of these foods will keep a person on the program, fine. Vegetable juices should still be the focus and the bulk of every meal.

"Every meal? Even breakfast?"

Look, folks. For breakfast, you drink hot bean extract (coffee) and eat undeveloped bird embryos (eggs) and the ripened ovaries of trees (fruit). You eat the muscles of ground-up pigs (sausage) placed between pulverized seeds fermented with a fungus (rolls), with a slice of curdled cow breast milk (cheese). And if I suggest vegetable juices, I'm the oddball?

So I conceded this and that to insure her compliance. Don't sweat the small stuff. After over a quarter-century as a quack, I know people.

Mrs. Kelremor's calls persisted for a while. At least I knew she was on the program. Over time, they were fewer and fewer. She seemed to be doing fine.

A year passed.

One day I was shopping in a friend's health food store. There were a few people at the checkout counter. One was a tallish lady—or, if not tall, she certainly had very good posture. "Remember me?" she said, with the unmistakable voice of Bela Lugosi on estrogen. I recalled only the voice. It did not match this graceful woman, at ease and smiling, buying a counterful of vitamins. But it was Mrs. Kelremor.

I greeted her, and she wasted no time in telling me, "I can work. I can bend, and reach, and sit and stand, and walk without any pain. I can work! I feel like a new woman." She actually said something more like, "I veel loke new voman," but enough of that.

I couldn't help but notice that the lumps on her arms and legs were gone. It wasn't surgery; a year and a half of juicing and vegetarian diet had apparently eradicated them. Now that was a bit unexpected. And all this progress, past age eighty.

37

Mrs. Kelremor is not the only person I know who juiced arthritis away. I saw something similar with a woman half her age.

The early forties is a bit young for rheumatoid arthritis, especially arthritis as severe as Cynthia's. Mostly I remember her hands. They were an old lady's hands. Swollen knuckles, fingers tightly drawn together to a point, almost like a paintbrush. Cynthia could hardly move them, and never without pain. The doctors, and there had been many, all told her that nothing could be done. Well, pain killers, but nothing else. Diet, perhaps? she'd asked them. Of course not, they'd told her.

She disbelieved them just enough to come and see me. I suggested that she do the same thing as Mrs. K had done, and hope for the same results. "And you are so much younger than her," I added. "Perhaps you have an advantage there."

At the very least, she complained a lot less. I had just one or two conversations with her on the phone after that. It was about eighteen months later when I actually saw Cynthia again in person. She had scheduled a follow-up appointment and breezed through the door into my office.

"Hi!" she said.

"Hello!" I answered. But who *are* you? is what I thought. Now I do not have a good head for names or faces to begin with, but this was extraordinary. I really thought there had been a mistake. I had gotten my appointment book messed up. This could not be Cynthia. I was expecting someone else, someone with at least some signs of arthritis.

This woman had none.

"Look!" she said. "Look what I can do!"

She flexed and turned her wrists and opened and closed all her fingers, effortlessly. I'm no orthopedist, but anyone could see that there was nearly complete range of motion.

"Wow!" I said. "What have you been doing?"

She looked at me as if I asked an odd question. "What we talked about," she answered. "I've been juicing every day, and fasting on juices every other week. For the last year and a half! And look at my complexion!"

Cynthia, or whoever this person really was, had almost no wrinkles. Her skin tone was perfect, perhaps a bit on the carotene-orange side. *USA Today* has described this harmless megajuicing side effect as looking like "an artificial sun tan." True. The doctors' *Merck Manual* describes hypercarotenosis as "harmless." Also true.

I describe it as "effective." There is more to juicing than just carotenes. The complex carbohydrates, raw food enzymes, minerals and vitamins, soluble fibers, and other vegetable nutrients makes for the perfect antidote to the protein-dominated, fat-heavy, sugar-laden, arthritis-causing Standard American Diet.

Once my own mother had arthritis. She was just entering her sixties. The symptoms were not severe, but they were getting worse each year. Then she started taking vitamins, juicing, and, most notably, eating lentil sprouts. Mom was a unique person, a "strange bird" as our old hardware-store man used to say. She will stick to an idea, even an untenable one, for a long time. This time, her talents for stubbornness were put to good use.

Every morning, Mom would have a large bowlful of sprouted lentils. Lentils look like brown split peas. To sprout them, she soaked dry lentils overnight in tap water. The next morning, she poured off the soaking water, then rinsed and drained them. Later that day, she rinsed and drained the lentils once more. They were ready for breakfast the next day. This may already sound pretty funky, but she went one step further: she topped them with molasses and ate them with a spoon.

Yum.

Now where does an otherwise intelligent person pick up ideas like this?

Guilty as charged. C'est moi.

I will stand on the results, though. I knew this lady and her hands especially well. It was considerably less than a year and my mom had no trace of arthritis. The raw sprout program worked. Juicing worked for Cynthia and Mrs. Kelremor. It all sounds quacky, because it is.

But that's how arthritis was eradicated from three sets of hands. To try it for yourself, start on "Saul's Super Remedy," as outlined in the beginning of Part Two.

Some illnesses are perceived as much harder to treat than they really are. Asthma, surprisingly, is a good example. The rule to remember is: Always consider the easiest and safest options first.

Six Ways to Avoid an Asthma Attack

1. **Take more C**. Low levels of vitamin C may cause asthma. High doses of vitamin C relieve asthma. "Decreased preference for foods containing vitamin C and decreased concentrations of vitamin C in blood plasma are also associated with asthma," says the *American Journal of Clinical Nutrition.*

   Robert Cathcart, M.D., recommends a daily vitamin C dosage of between 15,000 to 50,000 mg, divided into eight doses. He writes, "Asthma is most often relieved by bowel-tolerance doses of ascorbate. A child regularly having asthmatic attacks following exercise is usually relieved of these attacks by large doses of ascorbate. So far, all of my patients having asthmatic attacks associated with the onset of viral diseases have been ameliorated by this treatment." I have seen this work again and again. See my chapter "Vitamin C Megadose Therapy" for guidelines.

   When consumed in regular, frequent, near-saturation-doses, vitamin C is a powerful antihistamine. More on this in my chapter on allergies.

2. **Smoking** around asthmatics is assault, and smoking around children is child abuse. Smoking, or simply breathing second-hand tobacco smoke, destroys vitamin C. Don't smoke! And do not allow asthmatics near smokers. This goes double for children. It will not surprise anyone to learn that many scientific studies confirm the link between exposure to tobacco smoke and increased incidence of asthma.

3. **Reduce stress**. Stress reduction greatly helps asthmatics. See my chapter "Stress Reduction."

4. **Keep your back in line.** For you, this may mean regular visits to a good chiropractor. For me, it means yoga stretches, exercise, and using a "Ma" roller every day. Explanations and instructions can be found in the backache chapter.

5. **Avoid dairy products and meat**. Eat a lot of fresh, raw foods such as salads and fresh fruit. This is a tried-and-true naturopathic protocol.

6. **Look into homeopathic remedies**. I'd start with *aconitum napthallus,* a microdilution of the monkshood herb. It is good first aid for an asthma

attack. Taking lots of vitamin C will negate your need for even this natural remedy, however.

Recommended Reading

Browne GE, et al. Improved mental and physical health and decreased use of prescribed and non-prescribed drugs through the Transcendental Meditation program. Age of Enlightenment Medical Council, Christchurch, New Zealand; Heylen Research Centre, Auckland, New Zealand; and Dunedin Hospital, Dunedin, New Zealand (1983).

Cathcart RF. Vitamin C, titrating to bowel tolerance, anascorbemia, and acute induced scurvy. *Medical Hypotheses* 7 (1981): 1359–1376. (This paper is available to read in its entirety at www.orthomed.com.)

Graf D and Pfisterer G. Der Nutzen der Technik der Transzendentalen Meditation für die ärztliche Praxis. *Erfahrungsheilkunde* 9 (1978): 594–596.

Honsberger RW and Wilson AF. The effect of Transcendental Meditation upon bronchial asthma. *Clinical Research* 21 (1973): 278 (abstract).

Honsberger RW and Wilson AF. Transcendental Meditation in treating asthma. *Respiratory Therapy: The Journal of Inhalation Technology* 3 (1973): 79–80.

Kirtane L. Transcendental Meditation: A multipurpose tool in clinical practice. General medical practice, Poona, Maharashtra, India (1980).

Stone I. *The Healing Factor.* New York: Grosset and Dunlap, 1972.

Wilson AF, Honsberger RW, Chiu JT, and Novey HS. Transcendental Meditation and asthma. *Respiration* 32 (1975): 74–80.

"I've got a weak back."
"How long have you had it?"
"Oh, about a week back."
FROM AN OLD VAUDEVILLE ROUTINE

There is nothing like comfortably walking straight as a ramrod, proud to be bipedal. If you have back problems, there are two ways to achieve this. One is via a visit to a good chiropractor. The other is to use the techniques below. (*Important caution: common sense dictates the need of genuine care in dealing with any back problem. Consult a medical, osteopathic, or chiropractic doctor before proceeding with these, or any other, self-care approaches.*)

1. First, you can try some **bed stretches**. There are two ways to do them:

   Method One: Sit in the middle of the bed, legs straight out in front of you. Then, from the hips up, bend to the right as far as you reasonably can. Now lie back. You should be shaped like a boomerang, mate. And you will feel a profound "pulling" sensation in your lower back, hip, and upper leg. Relax and stay in that position for five minutes. Repeat the process to the left.

   Method Two: Lie across the bed face-down. Put your feet over the edge and grab the mattress with your toes. You can do this even if you are not an orangutan. While keeping your feet together, bend your upper body to the right as far as comfortable. You now will look like the other side of a boomerang. Using your arms, give it an extra stretch further to the right and hold it for a minute or two. Relax, and repeat for the left side.

   Both of these techniques work best if done first thing in the morning and last thing before going to sleep at night.

2. When you sleep, do so on a good, **firm (but not hard) mattress**. If you cannot afford a good mattress, consider asking Santa for a futon (a thick floor mat). You can also try putting a board under your lousy mattress for the time being.

3. Do back-healthy **exercises**. Try regular (or even irregular) practice of hatha yoga postures. Especially helpful are the Plow and the Hurdle Stretch.

   The Plow begins with a shoulder-stand on a well-carpeted floor. That's like a headstand, only your weight is on your shoulders, with your head tucked in and your bent arms propping up your back. I cannot do a real headstand, but I can do this. From the shoulder-stand, let the weight of your legs pull your feet to the ground directly behind your head. You will look and feel like a number 6 tipping over. Hold for the count of twenty, then do it again. And once more. This is a terrific before-you-hit-the-hay exercise.

Hurdle Stretches are easy to do. Sit cross-legged wearing loose clothing. Extend one leg out at a natural 45-degree angle from your hips. Reach down along that leg as far as you are able, drop your head, and reach a bit further. If you manage to reach your ankles, grab them and relax. If you can't, grab what part of your leg you can and relax. Hold with a slight stretch for the count of twenty-five. Repeat with the other leg. Repeat this several times, morning and evening, for best results.

Really want to feel great? Do some back-building, soreness-squelching exercises:

Shrugs. These are as easy as they sound. Simply shrug your shoulders—with a dumbbell in each hand. You can usually use quite a lot of weight for this. Beginners may want to start with five or eight pounds per hand. I use twenty-five-pounders, but then I've been doing this for a while. Your basic up-and-down shrugs can be complemented with shoulder rotations forward together and then backward together. Also, try alternate-shoulder up and down shrugs. These moves really loosen up the neck, shoulders, and upper back.

Flys. Use a *much* lighter weight for these. A fly is like a theatrical, expansive yawn with weights in your hands. Another way to describe flys is you look like a large bird stretching its wings, or Batman displaying his entire cape. Stand where you have a lot of free airspace around you and try some. By varying positions (one arm reaching up, the other down; both up or both down; reaching behind you backhanded; etc.) you can de-stress the entire upper half of your body to an extent you might not have thought possible. Start with a few and work up to either a larger number of repetitions or to larger weights. You can also hold heavier weights close to your body, with arms bent like a chicken dancing, and repeatedly stick your elbows back as far as they will happily go. Hey, this book is called "Doctor Yourself," not "Look Cool Doing It."

Side Crunches. Lie down on a carpeted floor in the good old "knee bent for sit-ups" position. But there's a twist: let both your knees fall to one side and do your crunches side-saddle. Do an equal number with your knees to the other side, of course. By bringing your knees nearly up to your chin, or extending your bent legs to one side or the other, you will feel a lower back benefit in addition to that most satisfying spare-tire-reduction that crunches are known for.

If you do a set of yoga postures or warm-up exercises first thing in the morning and again at bedtime, you will work better, sleep better, and feel better. Do this every day, and you will notice that you are able to reach further and touch those toes again. My high school phys ed teacher told me a long time ago that the single, simplest test of a person's physical fitness is to see if they can touch their toes. Can you? If not, do stretches. If you can touch them, continue doing stretches.

You can read even more on exercise in my chapter "Evading Exercise."

4. **Lose excess weight**. If you are twenty-two pounds overweight, that is like carrying a big economy-size bag of dog food around with you all day. Forty-four pounds is two big bags of dog food. All that weight pulls on your back and sits on your sacroiliac. Be realistic; it has to go. If you cut down your daily calorie intake by just 120 calories (a puny amount and you know it), you will lose a pound a month. If you do any exercise at all, you will triple the loss easily. Do not scoff at a monthly three-pound weight loss. That's thirty-six pounds in a year.

5. **Use a "Ma" roller**. A "Ma" roller is a wooden self-massage tool shaped something like a large, skinny spool. The twin raised sections toward the center deeply massage the back on either side of the spine. The sensation it produces resembles a full-back acupressure treatment by a barefooted lover. With patient, regular use, you can actually feel back bones slip into place. I have no financial connection with the manufacturer of this product. You can purchase one over the Internet or likely at your local health food store. They cost about the same as a single visit to a chiropractor. I have had mine for more than twenty years and use it every night before going to sleep.

6. **Fast, Totally Free, Utterly Effortless, Back-Friendly Advice:**

Ladies, stop wearing high heels. Nothing wrecks your posture and all the muscles and bones associated with it like walking around on your toes all day.

Lift, shovel, or rake with your "other" side. This really works. I learned it watching my dad, who one day picked up a large TV set with his left hand. His back went out and he was in considerable discomfort until he reached down and picked up the same TV with the other hand—and put his back "in" again. I used to get a backache after snow shoveling, a common event around these parts (I live just south of Canada). Then, I started shoveling backward. By this, I mean that I reversed the position of my hands on the shovel, dug to the other side, and threw with the other shoulder. This was weird at first, and I could only move a quarter of my usual load. But practice makes perfect, and now I have forgotten which side is my "other" side. I can move a ton of snow (literally) without injury. If you have no snow to move (you lucky person you), may I mention that this technique applies to shoveling dirt, concrete, manure, or anything else you have to toss about.

Wear that purse or backpack on the "other" shoulder. Same idea as above.

Make a point to periodically **notice your sitting posture**, whether working, reading, or watching TV. Can you improve it? Of course you can, once you become aware of it.

I know an unusually large number of chiropractors. This may be because I used to teach at a chiropractic college. One of my very best friends, Kenneth Hack, is an excellent chiropractor. He has "straightened out" my whole family for many years and he is great at it. But Ken lives too far from me for quick visits every time by back bugs me. So I have learned how to take care of it myself. I don't care much for exercise, but I exercise anyhow. Ken told me I have to, and I found out he was right. Good chiropractors teach you how to not need them. So now I do all the stuff I discussed above almost daily, because when I'm done, I feel terrific.

You can take this considerably further if you want to. Twenty-five years ago, I learned a gentle first-aid technique, "spontaneous release by positioning," developed by Lawrence Hugh Jones, D.O. Step-by-step instructions are provided in the next section.

Backache is a common ailment, one of the most common of all chronic health problems. It is certainly one of the chief on-the-job time-loss injuries. Most people will suffer backache at least some time in their lives. But the procedures described above are powerful steps you can take to prevent, and to relieve, backache.

I used to have back trouble. Now I don't.

Backache First Aid

One of the handiest techniques for putting annoyingly out-of-place vertebrae back into line (or "putting your back in") is called "spontaneous release by positioning." The technique was developed by Lawrence Hugh Jones, a Canadian doctor of osteopathy (D.O.). Dr. Jones published his technique in *The D.O.*, January 1964, pages 109–16. It is a very effective, noninvasive procedure that most anyone can learn and use.

Important caution: Common sense dictates the need of genuine care in dealing with any back problem. Consult a medical, osteopathic, or chiropractic doctor before proceeding with this or any other self-care approach.

Ironically, the very first time I had occasion to require spontaneous release was while I was taking a short course in how to do it. I really wasn't at all convinced of the value of the technique until it was used on me. This is so often the way, isn't it? One day I stepped off the curb to cross a street and suddenly felt my back give way and my leg get weak. I must have moved just right—or should I say, just wrong—and it threw my lower back out severely. I tried assorted exercises at home to try to correct it, but none worked. It was painful in the big muscles of the lower back, the lumbar area, and I couldn't do anything about it. So the next class, I asked the instructor to use me as the example of the day.

I was told to relax, and was rolled up into a ball with my leg up under my chest in an odd but strangely comfortable position. I knew that the teacher was pressing a trigger point beside my lower vertebra, but I only knew he was pressing the point because he told me he was. I felt no pain at all in this position—and believe me, that was amazing after my recent discomfort. A couple of minutes of relaxation passed, and he brought

45

my posture back to normal. The pain was gone, and it did not return. I rested a moment and got up and about again. I've been successfully employing spontaneous release ever since because it is gentle and it works so well.

"Spontaneous release" is another phrase for "nature cured it," applied to your back. Occasionally, a slightly displaced vertebra will slip back into place on its own. An unusual sleeping position or a chance movement can return a vertebra to its place, though not quite as easily as it can be put "out." This spontaneous realignment of the spine is not to be confused with "learning to live with it" or any other mere toleration of the aches or pains resulting from misplaced bones. It is one thing for the body to compensate for a problem, and quite another for the body to actually correct the problem.

So why is a technique needed at all if the body corrects itself? First of all, spontaneous release rarely occurs on its own. It would be nice if it did, but legions of backache patients prove otherwise. It seems easier for a bone to go out than to go in, in the same manner that it's easier to break a watch than fix it, or easier to scramble an egg than to put it back together again. Entropy rules, at least in this universe. When a bone goes out, the surrounding muscles also are affected. Dr. Jones explains this well in his paper. It seems that once the bone is out, the tendency of the muscles is to hold this new position. It's only through a unique position coupled with muscle relaxation that the bone can slip back into place almost unnoticed.

This is precisely what "spontaneous release by positioning" seeks to accomplish: this technique recreates the body's posture or position that put the vertebra out in the first place, to encourage it to replace itself of its own accord. It's like retracing your steps looking for your lost car keys.

By carefully positioning the arms or legs up or down, back turned this way or that, hips or neck pivoted right or left, a patient with even severe back pain will all at once find a comfortable position, a position where there is no pain, or almost no pain. It may be quite an odd-looking position, but the discomfort is eased or completely gone. This is the posture that encouraged the bone to go out in the first place; now we'll use the same position to encourage the bone to return. You can always tell when you've discovered the correct position because the patient will be comfortable, even if previously she was barely able to sit or stand. The very posture that put the initial strain on the back is now taking the strain off the back. Says Dr. Jones:

Even the severest lesions will readily tolerate being returned to the position in which lesion formation originally occurred, and only to this position. When the joint is returned to this position, the muscles promptly and gratefully relax. These joints do not cause distress because they are crooked; they are paining because they are being forced to be too straight. This is the mechanism of strain. (p. 110. Reprinted with permission of the American Osteopathic Association.)

In other words, the muscles are "used" to the strain, and contract to hold the bone out of place. When the person tries to straighten up, the bones won't, because the muscles won't let them. And the muscles won't relax because the bones are out of alignment. That is why heating pads, rubs, medicines, and "learn to live with it" do not solve the problem. Because those approaches do not reposition the bone, the muscle cannot relax to normal. That's why there's pain.

How to eliminate the pain? Reposition the bone back to normal. How? Return the person's body to the extreme but now comfortable posture so the muscles will relax. Then, hold the person in that position, as the person relaxes, for ninety seconds. Then, keeping the person relaxed, bring him back around slowly to a normal posture. The bone that was out will have returned with the rest of the spine to the normal position.

To better find exactly which vertebrae are out, and also to demonstrate to yourself that the bones do in fact realign and pain does disappear, it may be helpful to utilize what are called "trigger points" along the spine. Looking at the back, one can see the spinal column as a stack of bumps. To either side of each bump will be a trigger point. The distance out from the bump will be about one to two inches. Dr. Jones describes specific trigger locations in detail in his paper, and tells how to use them individually.

Each vertebra has side projections, like wings. If a given vertebra is misaligned, the tissue on one or both sides of that bone will be tender. This is because the bone's somewhat twisted condition strains the musculature and may even put pressure on the nerve emerging to each side of it. If you press there, it may hurt quite a bit. That's how you can tell which bones are out. Gently go up and down the spine and press lightly about one inch out to either side of each vertebral bump. Where there's pain, that's where the nerve is under pressure, where the muscle is locking, and where the bone is out. And that's the trigger point for that bone.

Generally, you'll find one side of the vertebra to be more tender than the other. In that case, keep pressing lightly on the tender spot while repositioning the person. When the correct position is reached, the person will say that he no longer feels pain even though pressure is still being applied on the trigger point. This is positive proof that you've found the right trigger point and the right position. Then, make sure the person is relaxing, hold the position while pressing the trigger point for at least ninety seconds, and then bring the person back to normal posture while continuing to press the trigger point. If you've corrected the problem, the person will not feel discomfort, and will not feel pain even though you continue to press the trigger point that hurt him before you started.

Summary of the steps of spontaneous release by positioning:

1. Find the right trigger point by gently pressing to each side of each vertebra. Pain indicates the trigger point.

2. While pressing that point, begin to reposition the person, asking him to tell you when the pain stops.

3. When a comfortable position is reached, continue pressing the trigger point while holding the person in that unusual position.

4. Be sure the person is relaxed if you want this to be successful. You, not the patient, must hold the position. If the patient holds the position, he is using the very muscles that you are seeking to relax.

5. After ninety seconds or more, return the person to a normal posture while continuing to press the spot.

6. If the person feels better and the trigger point pressure no longer hurts, then the bone is back in its proper place.

Step-by-step suggestions:

Step 1. The person's back should be uncovered. Some people will feel pain with only the lightest pressure to the trigger point. With other cases, you may have to press fairly hard to find the spot. Very muscular persons often require more pressure. Persons in great pain can require but a touch. I once worked on a relative whose back was in such excruciating pain that just a washcloth's pressure when taking a bath hurt him greatly. After half an hour of spontaneous release by positioning, he was so much improved that I could press those same spots on his back until my fingernails were white. That is real relief!

Step 2. Be sure to ask the person to tell you if a given trial position is better, worse, or the same. Some people won't tell you if you're helping or hurting, so ask! Ask constantly, "Better, worse, or the same? Better, worse, or the same?" If you're working on the neck, the person may begin in a sitting position. If you are working on the upper or middle back, the person might sit, or it may be easier to lie face down. For the lower back, the person may lie down on their side or face down. Start symmetrically and end symmetrically; that is, the patient should sit or lie straight to begin, and always end up straight with no crossed legs or slouching.

Step 3. The only comfortable position for the patient may be very unusual or extreme, and that's to be expected. The person may be in no pain at all only when rolled up like a ball, or twisted one leg over the other, or with their head pointed out and up with the chin in the air, or with their arm bent back over their shoulder! You just have to try any position until you get the sure sign that you've found the right one: no more pain.

Step 4. Dr. Jones mentions that "patients will try to help you. Don't let them." This is because spontaneous release by positioning must remain totally passive on the part of the patient; all he or she can do to help is to say when the pain is gone, and relax. That is it. After the procedure, the patient should rest for a while, and later endeavor to keep good posture while resting or working. This is important, because the bone replaced is most likely to slip back out of place if again offered the extreme position that did it before.

Step 5. The length of time that you have to hold the position will vary with each situation, from ninety seconds to as much as five minutes. Generally, the tenser the patient, the longer the hold time. Experience best shows how you can be the judge.

Step 6. With spontaneous release by positioning, as with math, you can always check your work. The trigger point that hurt when you pressed it showed you which vertebra was out; the trigger point when pressed with the person in the correct posture no longer hurt, so it showed you the correct position; the trigger point when pressed throughout the rotation of the person back to normal position no longer hurts, either, and shows you that the release was accomplished.

You cannot practice spontaneous release by positioning on yourself. You cannot have relaxed muscles if you are using them. You must exert force to position your limbs, or to press trigger points. You can either relax a muscle or use a muscle; you cannot do both together. This is why it is good to teach family members this technique: you may be the one needing it some day. If everyone learns, then you can help each other. When I did farm work, with much reaching, lifting, pulling, and carrying, my wife practiced spontaneous release by positioning on me almost every day. But she had her turn: when she was pregnant, particularly during the eighth and ninth months, I had to put her back in as much as twice a day. This prevented the considerable back discomfort that so many women complain of during pregnancy due to the extra weight applied to the back in carrying a child. (Gentlemen, you just try strapping one or two large bags of dog food around your middle and see how it feels!) All that new extra weight must be supported by the same bones.

Spontaneous release by positioning is my preferred way to relieve backache, and warm-up stretches or yoga postures are my preferred ways to prevent backache. See the previous section for directions on how to do those.

It still takes me aback (get it?) that there isn't more interest in spontaneous release by positioning from chiropractors or osteopaths. Maybe it is because the name is too long. Maybe it is because it takes more time than busy practitioners want to spend. Maybe it is because wellness self-reliance cuts into the profit of fee-per-visit professionals.

In other words, perhaps it is because the procedure works too well. This is a great technique. Help me spread the word.

Cancer

*It is common sense to take a method and try it. If it fails,
admit it frankly and try another. But above all, try something.*

FRANKLIN DELANO ROOSEVELT

Joe had terminal lung cancer, and no mistake. He was coughing up so much blood that he had a mostly red handkerchief in his hand all the while I talked with him in the living room of his small suburban home. Joe was too sick to come in to my office. In fact, he was too sick to get out of his recliner. In this chair his life played out, day and night. He could not walk. He was in too much pain to even lie down. He spent the night in his chair. He did not want to eat. But he did still want to live, and he was willing to try even vitamins if they would help him feel any better.

It was October and the leaves, orange and yellow, were falling outside the picture window as we talked. The TV was on, and some of the family was visiting. It is never easy to work with the dying. As a student, thirty years ago, I'd seen enough of them at the Brigham Hospital in Boston. Then, I had listened and watched. Now, I listened and watched and suggested vitamin C.

"How much?" Joe croaked.

"As much as humanly possible under the circumstances," I replied. I explained bowel tolerance to him, and answered the usual questions from the family. Most centered on how well it would work. Some were understandably skeptical; others were in overly optimistic denial. "If I had the sure cure for cancer, I'd be on the cover of *Time* magazine," I cautioned. "I can't promise anything, but vitamin C is very much worth trying, considering how sick Joe is."

All agreed that Joe had nothing to lose.

Here is what happened. Within days, Joe stopped coughing up the blood. If the C had done nothing else, this alone would have been more than enough benefit. But there was more good news within the week.

"Joe's appetite is back," said his wife. "And he is able to lie down in the bed now. He says he is sleeping much better and in much less pain."

Wonderful news, especially if you were Joe. Over and over I have seen terminal patients find profound pain relief and sleep improvement by taking huge doses of C. Again, if the C did nothing else, these benefits would be indisputable arguments for using it.

A week or so later, I heard still more news. "Joe is able to walk around the house with a cane. He's even walking around the yard!" His wife was quite emotional as she spoke. She knew, at some level, as we all did, that Joe was not likely to survive such severe cancer. And, in the end, he didn't. But he

50

extended his life, and the quality of that life was extraordinarily enhanced by the vitamin C. He never did all the other stuff I will recommend in this chapter; he couldn't. But he was determined to manage taking the C, and he did.

Oh, yes: how much did he take? About 4,000 mg every half hour he was awake, day or night. That is approaching 100,000 mg a day. He had a big jug of water, a big spoon, a big glass, and a big bottle of vitamin C crystals on the table right next to his recliner. And he never got diarrhea.

You may not believe vitamin C was responsible for the dramatic changes in Joe. I don't blame you—how could you, when you never hear about this stuff from your M.D.s? Rather, you tend to hear about natural treatments for cancer from sources dismissed as quacks, don't you?

Therein lies the problem.

For years, I've asked, "Who are the real quacks?" I've strongly implied, to say the least, that they are the conventional, tunnel-visioned sycophants of the medical, dietetic, and pharmaceutical professions. Not alone in this criticism, I quote endocrinologist Deepak Chopra, author of many a best-selling health book: "More people live off cancer than die from it." There is no profit in prevention, but plenty of money in disease. Like the firemen in Ray Bradbury's *Fahrenheit 451,* medical science encourages fires and then glamorizes their bungled attempts to put them out. By ignoring the evidence they don't like (and dismissing it as nonscientific), doctors and dietitians have closed the mausoleum door on millions.

Laetrile is a good case in point. This controversial anticancer agent, derived from almonds and apricot pits, has erroneously been called "vitamin B_{17}," but it is not a vitamin. Rather, Laetrile is amygdalin, a cyanide-containing substance. The cyanide is the active ingredient that somewhat selectively kills cancer cells—an action not unlike that of chemotherapy agents (which explains both the need for caution and the stringent rejection it has received from the medical powers that be). The imperious medical monarchy, which includes the AMA, FDA, and their ensuing laws, has made Laetrile therapy strikingly difficult to obtain inside United States borders.

Chapters 8 and 9 of Ralph Moss's *The Cancer Syndrome* disclose nitty-gritty details of some tantalizingly successful Laetrile research at Memorial Sloan-Kettering Cancer Center in New York City. It seems that experienced cancer researcher Dr. Kanematsu Sugiura repeatedly obtained lengthened survival time in mice with spontaneous mammary tumors. He also prevented tumors from spreading to the lungs and obtained temporary stoppage of small tumor growth. The problem is, he did all of this using Laetrile.

Dr. Sugiura's work constitutes limited, but nonetheless significant, findings. Sloan-Kettering's brass wanted him to shut up about the whole thing, and declared in press conferences that Laetrile had no value in cancer treatment. Once, Dr. Sugiura was personally addressed by a reporter, and he most expressly contradicted his bosses. How did author Ralph Moss know about all this? He was the number-two Sloan-Kettering PR man, that's how.

My personal view is that Laetrile is probably a palliative treatment, relieving suffering without necessarily obliterating the disease. Still, the fact that so many orthodox cancer foundations want it kept quiet is in itself sufficient reason to look into it more.

As the Laetrile example shows, there most certainly is a wider range of cancer treatment alternatives than conventional medical sources will allow. Worthy adjuncts and alternatives to chemotherapy, radiation, and surgical treatments are unpopular with organized medicine, yet are employed by far-thinking physicians and self-reliant persons around the world. Why is this? Because all possibilities need to be considered in undertaking the treatment of such a serious disease for which there are far too few survivors. In this chapter, I will let you in on some of the evidence that has accumulated and provide a natural protocol for adjunctive cancer treatment and prevention.

Vitamin C

Nobel-prize-winning scientist Linus Pauling, along with Ewan Cameron, a Scottish cancer surgeon, demonstrated the effectiveness of 10,000 mg of vitamin C a day in reversing terminal cancer in 13 out of 100 patients. These patients were given up as lost by medical authorities. Thirteen out of 100 may not seem like a high percentage of success, but keep in mind that those thirteen were considered beyond hope and then became free of the disease as far as could be determined. Thirteen is infinitely greater than zero. Vitamin C–treated patients lived, on average, five times as long as controls who did not receive the C. Do not be misled by false media hype against vitamin C. A pair of politically-motivated Mayo Clinic studies condemning the vitamin are seriously flawed. You will want to refer to Cameron and Pauling's book, *Cancer and Vitamin C,* for the full story. There is no substitute for the truth.

Of course 10,000 mg of vitamin C a day is greatly more than what the federal government maintains an average person needs. A reading of *The Healing Factor: Vitamin C Against Disease,* by biochemist Irwin Stone, will explain to you why we need so very much vitamin C, why it should indeed be normal to consume many grams of the vitamin a day, and why the lack of C is responsible for our species' present state of illness. Irwin Stone, by the way, is the person who got Dr. Pauling interested in vitamin C in the first place. For improved quality and length of life, the key is sufficient quantities of C. More orange juice just won't do it.

Opponents of vitamin C therapy would do well to acknowledge that Pauling and Cameron's work has been confirmed, perhaps most notably at Japan's Saga University by Murata and others (see "Recommended Reading" at the end of this chapter). Dr. Murata administered more than 30,000 mg per day and had even better results with terminally ill cancer patients. In the words of Dr. Louis Lasagna of the University of Rochester Medical School, "It seems indefensible not to at least try substantial doses of vitamin C in these patients."

There are many good reasons to give large quantities of vitamin C to a cancer patient. Ascorbic acid strengthens the collagen "glue" that holds healthy cells together and retards the spread of an existing tumor. The vitamin also greatly strengthens the immune system and provides a surprising level of pain relief.

But there is more. Vitamin C has been shown to be preferentially toxic to tumor cells. Laboratory and clinical studies indicate that, in high enough doses, one can maintain blood plasma concentrations of ascorbic acid high enough to selectively kill tumor cells. If you have not heard about this, it is probably because most of the best-publicized (but worst designed) vitamin C and cancer studies simply have not utilized high enough doses. Now, however, Hugh Riordan, M.D., and colleagues have treatment data which "demonstrate the ability to sustain plasma levels of ascorbic acid in humans above levels which are toxic to tumor cells in vitro and suggests the feasibility of using AA as a cytotoxic chemotherapeutic agent." See "Recommended Reading" for three of Dr. Riordan's studies.

These and many additional C-versus-cancer references may be obtained through your local library. A site search at my DoctorYourself.com website will also turn up a pile of them. You will want to request your librarian's assistance in locating some of the pioneering papers, such as those from the 1940s and 50s by William McCormick. His excellent "Have We Forgotten the Lesson of Scurvy?" and "Ascorbic Acid as a Chemotherapeutic Agent" are worth the search. Dr. McCormick shows that cancer symptoms and vitamin-C-deficiency symptoms overlap. The similarity between scurvy, which is obvious vitamin C deficiency, and cancer (particularly some forms of leukemia) is so great that it is incredible that billions of dollars of cancer research in the United States has failed to notice this.

Residential treatment for cancer by nutritional means has, for some time now, been readily available in Mexico, just south of the U.S. border. Odd, isn't it, that Americans have to flee the land of the free and home of the brave to get freedom of choice in cancer therapy? That's free trade for you. American medical doctor and nutritionist Frank Watts is one of a number of nonconformist physicians who have employed a therapeutic program that includes 20,000 mg of vitamin C daily plus Laetrile, vitamin A, vitamin B complex, and a strict vegetarian diet, among other things. In his experience, about 70 percent of six hundred terminal cancer patients have responded in some definite way to the treatment.

Precious few hospital-based megavitamin programs are available anywhere in the United States. Government and AMA pressure on doctors who advocate "megadose" vitamin therapy is high, research evidence notwithstanding. This will change, however, if citizens voice their views to the FDA, the AMA, the American Cancer Society, the National Cancer Institute, their lawmakers in Congress and state capitals, their insurance companies, and their own family doctors, and insist on unrestricted freedom of access to all options, including the unorthodox therapies, for cancer patients in this country.

While I'm at it, a caution. Beware of wolves in sheep's clothing: hospitals and other providers that offer so-called "holistic," "nutrition-based," "integrated," or "comprehen-

53

sive" therapeutic programs. The majority of them are only paying lip-service to consumers' requests for alternative cancer treatments, just to get them in the door. Their main approaches still tend to be chemo, radiation, and surgery. As a benchmark, first ask them if they give intravenous vitamin C, 30,000–100,000 mg daily. That'll settle out the mud in a hurry.

Other Vitamins

B-complex vitamins individually and collectively appear to be useful against cancer, in prevention as well as treatment. B-complex vitamins (as well as vitamin C) are water-soluble, easily-lost-under-stress vitamins. There is ever growing evidence that stress itself is a major factor in cancer—which makes sense, since stress depletes the body of B and C vitamins. Only in theory does the "balanced diet" that all of us are supposed to be getting every day supply ample quantities of these and all other vitamins. But no realistic allowance is made for the very real psychological and physiological demands that each person is daily subjected to. This is all the more true for a cancer patient.

In America, vitamin deficiency is the rule, not the exception. We are vitamin-deficient throughout our youth and even during gestation. According to *Nutrition Action Healthletter,* November 1993, researchers at the Children's Hospital of Philadelphia found that the mothers of children with cancer were less likely to have eaten fruits and vegetables, and were less likely to have taken multivitamins during the first six weeks of their pregnancy than mothers of healthy children. This resulting insufficient intake of folate, one of the B vitamins, appears to be a major cause of what are called primitive neuroectodermal tumors.

Vitamin B_6 has been found to be as effective, at least, as the drug usually used to treat recurrent bladder cancer, says *American Family Physician.* Many bladder patients are deficient in B_6. And they're not alone: 99 percent of adults nineteen and older get less than the RDA of B_6.

William McCormick cites researchers who found that cancer patients they tested were deficient in vitamin C by approximately 4,500 mg. When the RDA for C is 60 mg, is it any wonder?

It would be a tragic mistake to center any discussion of cancer on a single vitamin. Research will continue to confirm that all nutrients, and most certainly all the vitamins, are required to prevent and to stop cancer. After all, which wheel on your car can you afford to do without? Which wing on your airplane can we leave off next time you fly?

It is our population-wide but medically disavowed vitamin deficiency that is almost certainly the single most overlooked predisposing cause of cancer. We can either decrease stress or increase our vitamin supplementation, or preferably do both. Transcendental Meditation has been demonstrated to be clinically effective in both stress reduction and disease prevention. Research by David Orme-Johnson has shown that hospital admissions for benign and malignant tumors are less than half as common for long-time meditators. (See my chapter "Stress Reduction" for more information.)

If there were a drug that reduced tumors by 50 percent, you would have heard it proclaimed from the rooftops. Simple and natural tools are greatly underrated.

Nonvitamin Factors

Chlorophyll, the substance in plants that makes them green, may help control cancer by inhibiting cell mutations. Sprouts and the live food factors within them, such as enzymes and chlorophyll, have been extensively used by Dr. Ann Wigmore in nutritional programs to shrink or reduce tumors. The world's foremost authority on the anticancer properties of sprouts, wheat grass juice, fasting, and raw foods, Dr. Wigmore's lessons on the subject began with her Latvian grandmother and culminated with her self-cure of colon cancer using living foods. Her books include *Why Suffer?, Be Your Own Doctor,* and *Recipes for Longer Life.*

Zinc may also play a role in the prevention and treatment of certain forms of cancer. A study at MIT showed that animals fed a low-zinc diet are more likely to get cancer than those with normal diets. The majority of Americans do not get adequate zinc in their diets, either. There may even be a link between selenium intake and cancer. Parts of the country with selenium-rich soils have less cancer than selenium-poor-soil populations.

Of course, all these vitamin and mineral deficiencies are just aspects of the big problem: the overcooked, sugar-laden, meat-heavy diet we eat that got us into trouble in the first place. These "foods"—and other processed, worthless stomach fillers—are not good sources of what we need to live in health. Our national cancer epidemic is not a mystery. You don't have to just wait in line for a terminal disease with your name on it. There is much more to cancer prevention and therapy than the "food groups" and chemotherapy, radiation, or surgery. As much as these may help, there is at least as much good scientific evidence that nutritional alternative approaches to cancer work just as well or better. The essential cause of cancer most likely is many years of deficient diets.

Which means that the time to turn it all around is now, whether you have cancer or not. There is no need to wait for the AMA, the FDA, the *New York Times,* the American Cancer Society, or anyone else's approval. The safety margin with nutrients is enormous. Deficiency is what's dangerous. A determined patient, some good references and reading, an open-minded doctor, and the nutritional facts can do wonders. You may experience some difficulty in coming up with the open-minded doctor, but the rest is completely within your power. The following guide can help get you started. (*Commonsense caution: This is anecdotal information. Before embarking on any anticancer program, you should consult your healthcare provider.*)

Nutritional Support for Cancer Patients: A Typical Naturopathic Protocol

A. Digestive enzyme tablets

Two or more multiple digestive enzyme tablets per meal. The theory is that in cancer patients, the liver produces insufficient enzymes. Cancer patients eat and eat and eat but don't get the good stuff out of their food. They appear to be starving to death. Enzymes break down food so you can get the nourishment in it. A "multiple digestive enzyme" preparation is most efficient.

B. Kelp

3–5 kelp tablets per day. Kelp tablets are an iodine supplement. They have been reported to help resist healthy cell damage from radiation treatments.

C. Carrot juice

Begin by drinking at least one pint of carrot juice per day. Goal: up to two quarts (eight glasses). Raw food has lots of enzymes, and carrots are loaded with anticancer carotenes. About two pounds of carrots make one pint of juice. If possible, buy organic and buy in bulk. Look for economical twenty-five–pound bags because carrots keep fairly well. Select only fresh produce to get good-tasting juice. Yellow sprouts on carrots means they are old. Brush or scrape the carrots to clean them; there's no need to peel.

D. Green drink

Drink one glass (8 oz) green drink per day. Green drink is the freshly made juice of any green vegetable: celery, cucumber (peel to remove wax), green peppers, cabbage, broccoli, kale, lettuce (leaf, like romaine), whatever you find easiest to get down. Green drink is raw liquid chlorophyll, and chlorophyll and hemoglobin have curiously similar molecular structures. For green drink, do not use spinach, rhubarb, or beet greens. They contain oxalic acid.

E. B_{12} treatments

Either of the following will insure B_{12} absorption: intranasal B_{12} gel, paste, or spray, three times weekly; or weekly injections of 1,000 mcg. Ask for a prescription for the injections, or make your own intranasal B_{12} and save a fortune. See my chapter on B_{12} for directions.

F. Potassium

Potassium is in most fruits and vegetables. Carefully read the potassium chart ("K" stands for potassium) in Max Gerson's *A Cancer Therapy: Results of 50 Cases.* Eat no salt, and eat no "convenience" or canned foods, because they contain lots of salt. Cancerous cells love sodium, according to Dr. Gerson. More on the Gerson therapy in the next chapter.

G. Protein

Meat: Avoid it, especially red. Try to become a vegetarian. If you can't go all the way, fish is an excellent complete protein. Yummy recipe hint: Broil or bake fish, or poach it in half an inch of apple juice, simmering a few minutes on each side.

Tofu: Soy products contain cancer-fighting substances. Cut up some tofu into small pieces and throw it into whatever you are making. It will take on the flavor of the recipe.

Cheese: Natural, with no coloring added. Eat cheese if it will keep you off meat.

Yogurt: Low-fat, plain. Sweeten it yourself with a little fruit or honey.

Nut butters: Delicious and easy to digest. Buy them fresh and keep them in the fridge. Almond butter may inhibit the growth of tumors. Cashew butter is high in the amino acid tryptophan, which helps you sleep. With any nut butter, select the fresh, natural variety without added fat or sugar.

Milk: Speaking as a former dairyman, there is nothing like high-quality raw milk. I raised a family on it from infancy onward. Certified raw milk is inspected daily. Try to find it at a health food store or from a farmer. If not available, sweet acidophilus milk or watered-down yogurt digests better than pasteurized milk.

Sprouts: Eat two jarfuls per day. That is not a misprint. Sprouts are a complete protein, a complete food. A person could survive on a variety of sprouts and nothing else. Buy untreated seed. Alfalfa is a good one to start with, but also go for wheat and lentil. Toss in some mung bean, clover, cabbage, and radish sprouts for added flavor. Each day start two more jars. Harvest alfalfa at the end of 4–7 days; the others may be ready sooner. Wheat and lentil take only a day or two. Eat them in a sandwich or as the base for a salad. Dressings and garnishes are okay. Collect 12–15 wide-mouth quart jars and start farming. Ann Wigmore's books will tell you how to sprout, and why.

H. Fruits

Eat as many as you wish, any kind, any time. Before eating, wash them with soapy water, and repeatedly rinse.

I. Grains

Choose breads that are 100 percent whole grain. Read that label! Also, choose brown rice and whole-wheat pasta instead of their refined cousins.

J. Special Vegetables

Eat all the cauliflower, cabbage, Brussels sprouts, kale, and broccoli that you can. Research confirms that these cruciform vegetables are naturally rich in several phyto-chemicals that fight tumors. The other exceptionally fine food class is the legumes: peas, beans, and lentils. They are loaded with fiber, protein, minerals, and complex carbohy-drates. And they are really cheap. Eat lots.

K. Good Snacks

Fresh, unsalted popcorn is very healthy. On it, put 2 teaspoons nutritional yeast flakes, which give the popcorn a cheesy taste and additional B vitamins, chromium, and sele-nium. Raw veggies are the healthiest snack of all. Keep a tray of all your favorites in the center of your fridge, where you can reach it twenty-four hours a day. Celery, carrots, peppers, broccoli, cucumbers, tomatoes, and snap pea pods are all good choices.

L. Beverages

Vegetable juices, fresh and raw. (Whenever you cook, bottle, or can anything, the heat destroys its natural enzymes.) Other healthy drinks are fresh fruit juices, spring water or mineral water, herbal teas, and green tea or decaffeinated black tea.

M. Vitamins

Vitamins are concentrated nutrients. They are not drugs, so the safety margin is excellent.

Vitamin E: Begin with 200 IU of natural mixed tocopherols and gradually work up to about 1,000 IU daily. If you are on an anticoagulant drug (such as Coumadin), or if you are on medication for high blood pressure, your vitamin and drug doses probably will need to be tailored over a period of weeks. You can quite easily monitor your blood pressure at home, and your doctor can and should frequently check your prothrombin time for you. Occasionally blood pressure goes up slightly in folks not used to vitamin E. It is usually temporary. Reduce the vitamin E for a while, then resume a leisurely increase. If your "protime" gets too long, have your doctor reduce the drug dose, not the vitamin. Vitamin E greatly reduces the side effects of radiation therapy. Vitamin E is the body's number one antioxidant, very valuable in slowing tumor growth and slowing the spread of malignancies. You will very much want to read *Vitamin E for Ailing and Healthy Hearts,* by Wilfrid Shute, M.D., or any other book by him or his physician brother, Evan. They will walk you through the whole process.

Iron: If your physician says you need iron, take ferrous gluconate or ferrous fumarate iron tablets, which would substitute for your current prescription of harder-to-handle ferrous sulfate. Chelated iron tablets are better absorbed and, therefore, better utilized by the body. Iron is best absorbed if taken with vitamin C but not at the same time as vitamin E.

Vitamin C: Begin with 1,000 mg at each meal (3,000 mg per day). Your goal is bowel tolerance, which may be anywhere from 20,000–120,000 mg per day. It would be ideal to take some vitamin C every half hour you are awake, but that's a real nuisance. Do the best you can to divide the dose for maximum absorption. For stomach comfort at these high levels, buffering your vitamin C is strongly encouraged. Taking a calcium-magnesium supplement (any kind will do) along with the C is the simplest way to accomplish this.

For economy and a "fewer pills to take" feeling, try using vitamin C powder instead of tablets. Mix the powder in a sweet beverage such as fruit juice. Take the amount of vitamin C needed to feel better, to show improved lab tests, and to get well. Patients in remission should continue taking it for life. Do not be put off this valuable adjunctive therapy by unscientific scare tactics. Please be certain to read *Cancer and Vitamin C* by Ewan Cameron and Linus Pauling.

Carotenes and Lycopene: Until you get a juicer, you can do a lot with conventional cooked vegetables. Eat lots of yams, sweet potatoes, and winter squash. These are all very high in the natural carotenes, not just the best known beta form. Tomatoes, any way you like them, are loaded with lycopene, which is even more valuable than carotene. Do not let anyone keep you from your tomatoes with the old scare story that tomatoes are in the nightshade family and are therefore naughty. Bulgerdash. Tomatoes are good food. Studies in Italy (of course) showed that men who ate five to ten fresh tomatoes daily had almost no prostate cancer. Red or purple grapes (and other red/yellow/orange fruits and vegetables) are high in many other cancer-fighting antioxidants related to the carotenes.

Selenium: Only a minuscule amount is needed, generally around 300 mcg. A microgram is a millionth of a gram. Selenium works closely with vitamin E. Avoid excesses; more is not better in this case.

Zinc: The zinc in your multivitamin (perhaps 15 mg?) is low. Take 50 mg of zinc gluconate or preferably zinc monomethionine. Work up to perhaps 100 mg per day. Zinc reduces postsurgical healing time and profoundly strengthens the immune system. Take zinc with meals.

Calcium and Magnesium: Tablets can be used to conveniently buffer between-meal vitamin C doses. 1,500 mg of calcium and 500 mg of magnesium is a good target amount. Divide the doses as much as possible, including snack time and bedtime. Your body will absorb it much more efficiently that way.

Vitamin B Complex: Take one balanced B-50 tablet with each meal. If you are on intense drug therapy or are very fatigued, you can take additional B complex between meals with a snack. Patients on chemotherapy report greatly reduced nausea and much less hair loss when they take their B and C vitamins. You have to try this to believe it.

N. Suggestions

If you get diarrhea, ease up on the vitamin C or the vegetable juices. If not sure which, decrease one, then the other, to confirm the culprit. Bear in mind that diarrhea may be due to radiation or chemotherapy treatments. Cheese tends to help stop simple diarrhea. Chronic diarrhea requires medical attention.

If you need to sweeten something, try a little honey, sweet molasses, or pure maple syrup.

Give this protocol a full four-month trial, with 100 percent effort, before evaluating its success.

Don't eat anything without reading the label. Don't eat anything unless you know what it is. If you cannot pronounce it, don't eat it.

If your medical doctor is not familiar with orthomolecular (megavitamin) nutrition, hand him books, with the bookmarks stuck throughout, and ask, "Have you read what we've read?" Let Dr. Pauling and Dr. Hoffer and Dr. Riordan and Dr. Gerson and Dr. Cameron do the talking. When you go to battle, don't go without your best soldiers. If you are still unfamiliar with these physicians and their work, you are not ready to fight.

O. No-Nos

Sugar, smoking, and alcoholic beverages. (Organically produced red wine in moderation is a reasonable compromise. It is best to dilute it with two parts water before drinking. Better yet, drink grape juice.) Avoid artificial colorings and all preservatives. Do not consume aspartame (NutraSweet). Never eat any product containing saccharin, which has been found to cause cancer in laboratory animals.

Who gets the credit (or blame?) for this therapy? Certainly not me, although who wouldn't love to take the bow? But no, this is the collected, derivative work of many researchers. I'm not smart enough to come up with all this. I am just barely smart enough to find out who is getting good results . . . and copy them.

For more alternatives, spoken for by people who've had occasion to try them, it is well worth contacting members of The International Association of Cancer Victims and Friends (IACVF), The Gerson Institute, Alternative Cancer Treatments, or the Cancer Control Society. You will find up to date addresses and phone numbers at your public library or on the Internet.

Comfrey for Cancer

In an old issue of *Let's Live* (Oct–Dec 1958), H. E. Kirschner, M.D., wrote an almost unbelievable article about several important clinical uses of the comfrey plant (*Symphytum officinale*). Dr. Kirschner used comfrey in his medical practice to promote the healing of ulcers and wounds. He traces the history of comfrey back to 1568 and W. Turner's *Herball* which said "of Comfrey Symphytum, the rootes are good if they be broken and dronken for them that spitte blood, and are bursten. The same, layd to, are good to glewe together freshe woundes. They are good to be layd to inflammation."

He then cites Gerard's 1597 *Herball,* which indicated comfrey for ulcers of the lungs or kidneys, and Parkinson's 1640 *Theatrum Botanicum:* "The rootes of Comfrey, taken fresh, beaten small, spread upon leather, and laid upon any place troubled with the gout, doe presently give ease of the paines and applied in the same manner, giveth ease to pained joynts, and profiteth very much for running and moist ulcers, gangrenes, mortifications and the like."

Most significant is a citation from Tournefort's 1719 *Compleat Herbal,* which tells of one who "cured a certain person of a malignant ulcer, pronounced to be a cancer by the surgeons, and left by them as incurable, by applying twice a day the root of comfrey bruised, having first peeled off the external blackish bark or rind; but the cancer was not above eight or ten weeks standing." Even allowing for a possible misdiagnosis, this account is interesting.

Dr. Kirschner personally observed the powerful anticancer effects of comfrey on a patient of his who was dying from advanced, externalized cancer. He prescribed fresh, crushed-leaf comfrey poultices throughout the day. Much to the surprise of the patient and her family, there was obvious healing within the first two days of treatment, with continued visible improvement over the next few weeks. "What is more," he writes, "much of the dreadful pain that usually accompanies the advanced stages of cancer disappeared," and there was a dramatic decrease in swelling. Dr. Kirschner concludes by regretfully saying that the cancer had already spread to the inner organs "which could not be reached with the comfrey poultices, and the woman died."

Just in terms of quality of life, the degree of healing that *did* occur under the comfrey poultice treatment is of tremendous significance. Here is a "folk" remedy providing, at the very least, significant palliative relief, and to a remarkable extent reversing a cancerous growth. We can ill afford to overlook the full potential of external comfrey-leaf poultices to heal sores and wounds of all types, including burns and gangrene, as well as "tumors both benign and malignant," says Dr. Kirschner.

Taken internally as decoction (boiled root tea), comfrey is described as effective against tuberculosis, internal tumors, and ulcers, and promotes the healing of bone fractures. If it is hard to understand how one simple plant can be so widely useful in healing, remember that penicillin's supporters have made some pretty broad claims for the mold on oranges.

Dr. Kirschner describes in his article how to prepare comfrey leaves and roots for home use. The leaves are for external use, and the root for internal use. Anyone can grow comfrey in their garden. In fact, just try to stop this virtually indestructible perennial. As a young man, I decided to plant comfrey all over my yard. That took about fifteen minutes. It grew so vibrantly that I eventually decided to eradicate the comfrey. It took twenty years to root it all out. Well, most of it. There is still that patch over there on the side. . . . I got my "starter" comfrey from a friend, and now I know why he was smiling so broadly as he handed the huge sack of roots to me.

Comfrey is widely available. Ask around and see who's got some to share. Or try a garden supplier, nursery, or herb store. How to plant comfrey: stick the root under ground and come back in a month or two. To grow: stand back and watch.

To use the leaves, one simply picks them, crushes them into a nice emerald green paste, and applies topically. Although dried leaves are often available in herb and health food stores, it is much better to use fresh-cut leaves right from the garden.

Roots can be prepared by boiling one-half to one ounce of minced or crushed root in two cups of water. I thoroughly brush and wash the root under tap water before slicing it up. Then I place the chunks in the water in a glass or stainless steel pan. Bring it to a boil, continue boiling for five to ten minutes, and let sit until it is cool enough to drink. This *decoction* is much more effective than simply steeping in hot water. Dose: one six-ounce glass, several per day, as required. Fresh root is almost certainly best, but I expect that dried root retains some therapeutic value.

Caution: Herbs may be the most natural of medicines, but they are still medicines. There are potentially harmful side effects if nonboiled comfrey is consumed in appreciable quantity. This warning especially applies to what is sometimes called "comfrey-leaf tea," which I specifically advise you to avoid. In my opinion, pregnant or nursing women should decline to use any medicine. To be comfy with comfrey, consult your doctor and a reliable herbal textbook (such as John Lust's *The Herb Book*) before employing this, or any, herbal remedy. It is important to meet potential physician objections with a clear understanding of the "comfrey rule": *fresh leaves externally, boiled root decoction internally.*

Allantoin, a key ingredient found in abundance in comfrey, may be among the reasons comfrey works. Allantoin helps cells to grow and grow together. Since this is precisely what is needed for ulcers, tumors, burns, broken skin, broken bones, and perhaps even malignancy, it is little wonder that comfrey has a respect in folklore and medical practice throughout the world. For a definitive explanation of how, why, and what comfrey heals, with detailed information on the chemical constitution of allantoin, read a long-forgotten sixty-page work entitled *Narrative of an Investigation Concerning an Ancient Medicinal Remedy and its Modern Utilities* by Charles J. MacAlister, M.D., and A. W. Titherley, D.Sc. It is full of case histories, research, and historical information. Clinical observations, notes on malignancy, and instructions on how to prepare the remedy are included. This 1936 book is even rarer than Dr. Kirchner's article that I cited above. Reprints of either may still be available on microfilm. It is a good idea to ask your public library's interlibrary loan person to help you obtain copies.

Recommended Reading

Cameron E and Pauling L. *Cancer and Vitamin C,* revised edition. Philadelphia: Camino Books, 1993.

Dr. Harold W. Manner: the man who cures cancer. *Mother Earth News.* (Nov/Dec 1978): 17–24.

Hanck A, ed. *Vitamin C: New Clinical Applications.* Bern: Huber, 1982, 103–113.

Hoffer A. *Vitamin C and Cancer: Discovery, Recovery, Controversy.* Kingston, ON: Quarry Press, 1999.

Kulvinskas V. *Survival into the Twenty-First Century.* Wethersfield, CT: Omangod Press, 1975.

Moss R. *The Cancer Syndrome.* New York: Grove Press, 1980.

Moss R. *The Cancer Industry.* New York: Paragon Press, 1989.

Murata A, Morishige F, Yamaguchi H. Prolongation of survival times of terminal cancer patients by administration of large doses of ascorbate. *Int J Vitamin and Nutrition Res Suppl* 23 (1982): 103–113.

Orme-Johnson D. Medical care utilization and the transcendental meditation program. *Psychosom Med* 49 (1987): 493–507.

Pauling L. *How to Live Longer and Feel Better.* New York: W. H. Freeman, 1986.

Riordan HD, Jackson JA, Schultz M. Case study: high-dose intravenous vitamin C in the treatment of a patient with adenocarcinoma of the kidney. *J Ortho Med* 5 (1990): 5–7.

Riordan NH, Riordan HD, Meng X, Li Y, Jackson JA. Intravenous ascorbate as a tumor cytotoxic chemotherapeutic agent. *Medical Hypotheses* 44 (March 1995): 207–213.

Riordan N, Jackson JA, Riordan HD. Intravenous vitamin C in a terminal cancer patient. *J Ortho Med* 11 (1996): 80–82.

Stone I. *The Healing Factor: Vitamin C against Disease.* New York: Grosset and Dunlap, 1972.

Wigmore A. *Why Suffer?* New York: Hemisphere Press, 1964.

Wigmore A. *Recipes for Longer Life.* Garden City Park, NY: Avery, 1982. (All her recipes contain no cooking at all!)

Wigmore A. *Be Your Own Doctor.* Garden City Park, NY: Avery, 1983.

Williams RJ, Kalita DK, eds. *A Physician's Handbook on Orthomolecular Medicine.* New Canaan, CT: Keats Publishing, 1977.

Max Gerson was a medical genius who walked among us.
NOBEL-PRIZE WINNER ALBERT SCHWEITZER

Max Gerson, M.D., started his professional life as a distinguished physician and ended it condemned as a quack. This highly trained scientist turned his back on conventional medicine and never recanted.

The renegade doctor does not fit the public perception of quack very well. We want our quacks flaming, as Homer Simpson wanted all his gay acquaintances to be. Only a real nut of a quack, an utterly uneducated, criminally flamboyant fraud, is repellent enough to be sure to scare patients into the waiting arms of the drug doctors. Max Gerson is therefore a problem from the start, best left ignored. He was entirely too qualified, too experienced, and too radical. You will look long and hard for any positive reference to him in any medical history or textbook. And yet, this man developed the single most successful treatment for cancer in existence—more than sixty years ago.

Gerson was a surgeon in the German army during the first world war. He and other doctors worked MASH-like twenty-hour days, operating on what was left of their countrymen evacuated from the front lines. The British naval blockade of Germany had resulted in a dire shortage of morphine for patients in recovery. The doctors, who drank coffee to stay awake day and night to operate, found that coffee also relieved pain in the wounded. To this day, caffeine is one of the active ingredients in many an extra-strength pain-reliever. Some soldiers had so much of their faces, throats, and stomachs shot away that they were fed by rectum—not an uncommon practice in the old days. Desperate nurses were instructed to put coffee in the enema water of these individuals. It worked; any port in a storm.

This was the first reason why Dr. Gerson would later give coffee enemas to cancer patients: pain relief. He later claimed another: rectally administered coffee seemed to stimulate the liver to flush waste from the system. He was neither the first nor the last to believe that "accumulated toxins" are a cause of cancer. It is a persistent and recurrent quacky notion . . . which is also probably quite accurate.

The cancer-preventive aspects of high-fiber diets support this. One study showed that Hispanic women have far lower rates of breast cancer than do black or white women. When all factors were considered, only one difference could be found: Hispanic women eat considerably more beans than black or white women do. The fiber is almost certainly the secret. Other research has pointed to the flip-side conclusion: low-fiber diets are carcinogenic. In a low-fiber diet, any consumed carcinogens have a longer transit time through the body's digestive tract. More time in contact with the lining of the GI tract means more opportunity for carcinogenesis.

Lots of fiber may also help the body excrete excess endogenous chemicals, such as estrogen, thereby lowering the rate of some hormone-dependent cancers. Additionally, soluble fiber removes excess bile acids (by-products of fat digestion) that are also linked with cancer. David Reuben's *Save Your Life Diet* (yes, he was an M.D. as well) discusses fiber's anticancer roles in detail. That book came out in the 1970s; this is not new information. Why isn't it more widely known? Fiber is simply too cheap for any pharmaceutical company to make big bucks off it. There is more money in chemo than Beano.

The goal of the Gerson approach, which makes it the exact opposite of chemotherapy, is its attempt to detoxify the body, focusing on restoring and strengthening liver function. Is this a reasonable focus? Well, weighing in at about four pounds, the liver is the largest gland in the body. It is the body's site of detoxification of alcohol and other drugs, and could very well detoxify a cancer patient. If so, the liver may well be the key organ for cancer therapy.

To build up the body's ability to fight cancer, Dr. Gerson then employed the most damning therapy in the twentieth century: vitamins. On top of that, he was among the pioneers recommending extensive vegetable juicing. There you go: this all would be right at home on a shopping channel at 2 A.M.

Oddly enough, it was because he had chronic, severe migraines that Max Gerson got into vitamins and juicing. He found no help in the drugs of the day. Remember, he was a doctor and he well knew what was available. Nothing worked. So Gerson tried the logic of that great nonperson, Sherlock Holmes: if all reasonable explanations fail, the answer must be some unreasonable one. Immersed in the unreason that only pain can generate, Gerson tried different foods, doing an early version of what was probably much like allergy testing. He found that juiced vegetables, not medicines, were the cure for his headaches. He was as surprised as you would be, perhaps even more so, because he was a drug doctor who had been taught nothing of natural healing, except perhaps contempt for it.

Nothing succeeds like success. Word got around and people started to seek out this doctor who cured migraines when the other doctors failed to. Gerson began to note that many of his migraine patients were also getting cured of assorted conditions that they hadn't even initially told him about. He reasoned that juicing was a "metabolic therapy," nonspecific and broad in nature. If that concept annoys you, think of the diverse sicknesses that are expected to respond to a given antibiotic.

Up until this point, Gerson was not even thinking of treating cancer. When ultimately asked to try, he refused, having no intention of becoming known as another cancer quack. Pressure from suffering patients eventually changed his mind. He hesitatingly began using the metabolic therapy, cleansing and restoring the cancer patient's body, and was curing more than 50 percent of terminal cancer patients. This extraordinary success rate was in part the basis for a 1946 Congressional hearing on cancer therapies. Gerson took fifty of his carefully documented case histories before an investigative committee. Radiation, surgery, and chemotherapy were all approved for the "war on cancer." Vitamins, juices, and Gerson were excluded, by just a handful of votes.

Well, what do you expect? His mistake, and it was a big mistake, was to recommend coffee enemas for cancer patients. The fact that dying patients were recovering was secondary. It all sounded too quacky. The juices and the vitamins just added insult to injury. In the great traditions of Congress, they got it wrong and threw out the baby with the bathwater. Gerson remained a medical outsider for the rest of his life.

For over sixty years, cancer treatment and research has been almost entirely restricted to cut, zap, and drug: surgery, radiation, and chemotherapy. Billions and billions of dollars have been expended investigating every cure *but* a nutritional one. Ridicule, not science, has kept the Gerson therapy away from your local oncologist's office. Try a simple test: ask ten doctors what they think of using the Gerson therapy against cancer. Then ask the same doctors what they *know* of the Gerson therapy. I'll lay good odds that about all they know is that the guy used coffee enemas. "Would you like cream and sugar with that?" a physician once said to me. And you'll likely hear worse.

The best possible summation of Dr. Gerson comes from the great Nobel laureate Albert Schweitzer: "I see in Dr. Max Gerson one of the most eminent geniuses in the history of medicine. He has achieved more than seemed possible under adverse conditions. Many of his basic ideas have been adopted without having his name connected with them. He leaves a legacy which commands attention and which will assure him his due place. Those whom he has cured will attest to the truth of his ideas."

Recommended Reading

Gerson C and Walker M. *The Gerson Therapy.* New York: Kensington, 2001.

Gerson M. *A Cancer Therapy: Results of Fifty Cases and the Cure of Advanced Cancer.* San Diego, CA: The Gerson Institute, 2000.

Straus H. *Dr. Max Gerson: Healing the Hopeless.* Kingston, ON: Quarry Press, 2002.

Dysplasia is a study in scurvy. In vitamin C–deficiency disease, there is insufficient production of collagen, the strong, healthy glue that holds your cells together. Whether dysplasia is triggered by a virus, physical irritation, or other cause, the fundamental problem is weak intercellular ground substance due to inadequate ascorbic acid. William J. McCormick, M.D., addressed the basics of this subject in a series of papers more than forty years ago. (Specific vitamin C megadosage instructions are provided in the chapter "Vitamin C Megadose Therapy.")

Chronic dysplasia is sometimes feared to be precancerous. In addition to vitamin C, another major factor in preventing such an unwanted development is the amino acid L-lysine. I have seen physician reports that women who take several thousand milligrams of L-lysine daily get far less cervical cancer. While we await confirmation, there is no down side to eating foods high in L-lysine. This is because you can get lots of lysine by eating lots of beans. Beans, and all the other legumes, are loaded with lysine. Peas are very high in lysine. So are lentils, refried beans, pinto beans, kidney beans, three-bean salad, bean soup, bean burritos, veggie bean-burgers, and even chickpeas. Lima beans are relatively low in lysine; soybeans (and anything made from soy) are unusually high. An effective dose is about 3,000 to 4,000 mg of lysine daily. That is about a can and a half of beans each day.

Wait! Before you go off singing the "musical fruit" song, hear me out. I know you are going to ask, and I have an answer all ready for you:

Suggestions for Reducing Social Embarrassment after Following Saul's Bean Program

First, drain em! Do *not* use the liquid that canned beans are packed in, nor the water that you soak or cook beans in. Such processing liquid is high in raffinose sugars, which are gas-producing par excellence. Why? Because bacteria love them, that's why. Odoriferous gas is produced by bacteria in the large intestine as they munch on incompletely digested food. You will doubtless be pleased to know that most intestinal gas is odorless methane, odorless hydrogen, and odorless carbon dioxide. But then there's hydrogen sulfide (from bacteria eating protein) which the human nose can detect at just *one part per two billion*.

Odor also partly results from amines, which are formed by intestinal bacteria from amino acids (protein again). Eating less protein in general, and less flesh protein in particular, has an olfactory benefit. The stool of a cow is a lot less unpleasant than the stool of a dog. Since the average American eats two to three times more protein a day than is necessary, you need not worry about wasting away from reduced protein consumption.

Did you know that the average person forms 1 to 3 pints of bowel gas each day, with about fourteen emissions?

Did you know that this was one of the most quoted facts students lifted from my Clinical Nutrition lectures?

Okay, now for the "bottom" line.

GAS Rx

One: slow down and chew your food very well. Undigested starches are a major culprit in flatulence. The slower you eat and better you digest, the less of a problem you'll have.

Two: sprout your beans, or cook them thoroughly. Remember: drain off that canning or cooking water!

Three: allow time for intestinal bacteria to adapt to dietary changes. Most new near-vegetarians have a not-new body, full of stuff from the old days of revelry. Transition can take a while, but I think you will *feel* better right away. As your legume-lovin' bowel bacteria (and other good intestinal flora) begin to really thrive, you will barely notice that you have become a virtual dean of the beans. And that ever worrisome "crowded elevator syndrome" will also decrease dramatically.

Four: cut down on sweets. Excess simple carbohydrates are a good culture medium if you want excess bacteria, so put the little beggars on a diet.

Recommended Reading

Liebman, B. Out of gas? Center for Science in the Public Interests Nutrition Action Healthmatter, (March 1991).

McCormick, WJ. Cancer: The preconditioning factor in pathogenesis. *Archives of Pediatrics of New York,* 71(1954): 313.

McCormick, WJ. Cancer: A collagen disease, secondary to nutritional deficiency? *Archives of Pediatrics New York,* 76(1959): 166.

McCormick, WJ. Have we forgotten the lesson of scurvy? *Journal of Applied Nutrition.* 15(1,2) (1962): p. 4–12.

In an average lifetime, the human heart will beat two and a half *billion* times. But, as in Vegas, there is no guarantee that the odds will favor anyone. Congestive heart failure (CHF) is the end product of any of a number of cardiovascular diseases that degrade the heart's ability to pump blood efficiently. Much has been written on diagnosing CHF but rather less is known about treating it. This is because broken hearts are tough to fix. A diagnosis of CHF means that it is too late for nutritional prevention. The horse is long gone by the time most people decide to shut the stable door. But nutritional intervention can still greatly help a damaged heart.

In the past, drugs such as digitalis were often given to strengthen and to some extent regulate heartbeat. Vasodilators (blood vessel–opening drugs) are given to improve cardiac output and relieve backed-up blood from blood vessels throughout the body, especially in the lungs. Fluid buildup (edema) is commonly treated with diuretic drugs.

It may be possible to naturally augment, or perhaps substitute for, these pharmaceutical drugs. The following is a protocol that can be tried under the auspices of a qualified health practitioner.

Vitamin E

One of the body's most powerful defenses against free-radical damage is the antioxidant vitamin E. The natural form, d-alpha-tocopherol, can also be cautiously used to strengthen and regulate heartbeat. To avoid any possible risks of an asymmetric heart contraction, patients with CHF need to start small with vitamin E. An initial dose of vitamin E should be only about 50 IU daily. This is roughly equivalent to 50 mg. Doses may be gradually increased under medical supervision. For additional information, it is most worthwhile to read any books by Wilfrid or Evan Shute. Their books are often hard to find, so try an interlibrary loan at any public library.

Thiamine

Some CHF is actually caused by thiamine (vitamin B_1) deficiency. 25–50 mg with each meal will overcome any such deficiency. I think a thiamine-containing 50 mg "balanced B complex" tablet each meal would be even better.

Common Sense

No added salt. No alcohol. No smoking. No extra weight. No kidding.

Herbal Diuretics

It may be possible to use herbal medicines to reduce swelling due to retained fluids. There are no fewer than 180 herbs with diuretic properties listed in John Lust's *The Herb Book.* I am not suggesting that you take 180 herbs. I am suggesting that you read up on your options before committing yourself only to drugs.

Selenium

Selenium deficiency can cause a congestive heart disease called Keshan disease. 100–300 mcg of selenium daily will insure against this. In addition, selenium works to help your body recharge and efficiently reuse its vitamin E.

Magnesium

The role of magnesium in normal heart function is tremendous. Profound magnesium deficiency causes muscles to malfunction or not function at all. Several hundred of your body's most important biochemical reactions depend on this mineral, including the synthesis of proteins, DNA, fats, and carbohydrates. Even most, ah, "healthy" adults fail to get the RDA of magnesium, which is about 400 mg. These figures are elemental weights: just the corn, not the can. Most magnesium supplements are compounds of magnesium with something else. The weight of the "something else" is often obscured in dosage recommendations. That is why Melvyn Werbach cites studies that advocate daily dosages of 2,000 mg of magnesium compound per day for CHF in his *Textbook of Nutritional Medicine.* The elemental quantity is significantly lower than that. Green vegetables and whole grains contain quite a bit of magnesium. Pinto beans, almonds, and especially figs are other outstanding food sources.

Of the oral supplements, magnesium aspartate or magnesium orotate may have the best chance of getting into cardiac muscle cells. These forms of magnesium are rarely found on store shelves. Your doctor may be able to have them compounded for you by a cooperative pharmacist, or you might find them with an Internet search. Intravenous administration of magnesium may be necessary in more serious cases of CHF. Have a test ordered to check serum magnesium. Most doctors don't. It is even better to check myocardial magnesium. This is because the amount of magnesium in the heart muscle cells may be considerably lower than that in the blood.

Potassium

Potassium deficiency is associated with CHF, and is connected with magnesium deficiency. Low potassium can cause erratic heartbeat (heart arrhythmia). A very safe and very easy way to increase dietary potassium is to eat lots of easily digestible fruits and juiced vegetables. They are loaded with potassium. Nuts, whole grains, and legumes are good, too. Four ounces of almonds contains a whopping 800 mg. Brazil nuts have almost as much.

Coenzyme Q_{10}

Coenzyme Q_{10} increases energy, probably due to its role in facilitating cellular respiration in the mitochondria of heart muscle cells. One of the best things about Coenzyme Q_{10} is that it is harmless, having no negative side effects or contraindications of any kind. No physician or hospital can make a case against taking it. The down side is that it is pricey. But then, so are heart transplants. Clinical studies and patient reports that show success with CoQ_{10} usually use somewhere around 400 mg a day, divided into several doses. 35 or 50 mg per day simply will not work.

I have read physician reports asserting that after regularly taking CoQ_{10}, patients with severe CHF (so severe that they were waiting for a heart transplant) no longer needed the operation. I can't imagine higher praise than this.

Amino Acids

As a rule, I am in favor of getting amino acids through the protein in one's diet. With really sick people, however, a case can be made for amino acid supplementation. Dr. Werbach recommends L-arginine at a daily dose of 5,600–12,600 mg because it opens peripheral blood vessels and raises the heart's output. Patients given the supplement found they could walk longer, due to the improvement in blood flow while exercising. Arginine is normally considered by dieticians to be a "semiessential" amino acid, necessary only for growth. But growth may well include regrowth, strengthening, and repair of cardiac muscle. Eggs, cheese, whole grains, and legumes are good food sources. Peanuts are absolutely loaded with arginine, containing three times as much as meat does. You'd need to consume roughly a twelve-ounce can of peanuts a day to get in the middle of the dose mentioned above. That, or consider supplements. Chew nuts well for best absorption.

Taurine is an amino acid normally made in your body from another amino acid, methionine. Methionine is found in eggs, cheese, beans, nuts, and whole grains. Brazil nuts have over twice as much methionine as meat, ounce for ounce. Extreme stresses to the body (hospital food, perhaps?) can cause taurine deficiency. Taurine appears to help regulate heartbeat. Dr. Werbach recommends a dosage of 4,000–6,000 mg per day.

The amino acid L-carnitine is also made in your body *if* (and, to misquote Ed Sullivan, this is a "really big" if) you consume plenty of the amino acids methionine and lysine, and vitamin B_6, niacin, and vitamin C. Most people, especially the elderly suffering from chronic illness, do not get nearly enough of these vitamins. One study recommends 2,000 mg of L-carnitine daily for CHF.

Large amounts of supplemental creatine, still another amino acid that your body normally produces, may help strengthen heartbeat. As creatine phosphate, it is involved in supplying energy to power muscle tissue, especially cardiac muscle. Dr. Werbach cites studies indicating that persons with CHF have a deficiency of creatine in the heart muscle itself, and that daily doses of 20,000 mg per day improve cardiac function, physical strength, and endurance.

All quantities mentioned above should be divided up into several smaller doses throughout the day. I would add vitamin C, ranging anywhere from 4,000–10,000 mg per day all the way up to bowel tolerance. C is vital because of its antioxidant properties and because of its role in connective tissue synthesis. I also suspect that since the heart prefers fatty acids for fuel, a long-standing deficiency of essential fatty acids causes deterioration of heart muscle. Lecithin, fish, and primrose oil are sources of essential fatty acids.

If these natural options do not speak strongly enough to you, bear in mind that:

1. There is no drug cure for congestive heart failure; and

2. The pharmaceutical drugs given in an attempt to cope with the condition have many side effects; and

3. The National Institutes of Health have issued some depressing statistics about CHF:

> "Nearly 5 million Americans have CHF, and half of the patients diagnosed with CHF will be dead within five years. Each year, there are an estimated 400,000 new cases. And CHF is the most common diagnosis in hospital patients age sixty-five and older.
>
> Incidence of CHF is equally frequent in men and women, but survival following diagnosis of congestive heart failure is worse in men. Even in women, only about 20 percent survive much longer than twelve years. The outlook is not much better than for most forms of cancer. The fatality rate for CHF is high, with one in five people dying within only one year. CHF remains a highly lethal condition.
>
> An ideal CHF therapy would be to improve the heart's pumping ability, open clogged arteries, and prevent tissue damage from free radicals, a byproduct of the body's metabolic processes." (Data Fact Sheet: Congestive heart failure in the United States: a new epidemic. U.S. Dept of Health and Human Services, Public Health Service, National Institutes of Health, National Heart, Lung, and Blood Institute, September 1996.)

Most people appear to have found very little reason to believe that there are serious options for people with this serious disease.

But there are.

Recommended Reading

Data Fact Sheet: Congestive heart failure in the United States: a new epidemic. U.S. Dept of Health and Human Services, Public Health Service, National Institutes of Health, National Heart, Lung, and Blood Institute, September 1996.

Desai TK, et al. Taurine deficiency after intensive chemotherapy and/or radiation. *Am J Clinical Nutrition* 55 (1991): 708.

Ghidini O, Azzurro M, Vita A, Sartori G. Evaluation of the therapeutic efficacy of L-carnitine in congestive heart failure. *Int J Clinical Pharmacology, Therapy and Toxicology* 26 (1988): 217–220.

Werbach M. *Textbook of Nutritional Medicine.* Tarzana, CA: Third Line Press, 1999, 273–275.

Ever since I got a letter from a woman who wanted instructions for doing her own thoracic surgery—by correspondence—I have more truly realized the need for absolute clarity in writing a section like this one. So here it is: I am not utterly opposed to using the valid skills of well-trained medical professionals. Get a physician's opinion first, of course. There are limits to what you can do. (By the way, I told the woman to see a surgeon. I considered suggesting that she also see a psychiatrist.) Yet there are many things we can do for ourselves—and arguably better than a harried, hurried, hired practitioner.

I offer for your consideration (as Rod Serling would say) one or two of my more delightful childhood medical dramas, or should I say, traumas.

As kids, we were always building something in the woods behind my parents' house. After we built our tree fort (as differentiated from a mere tree house, mind you), we practically lived there. As work gloves were for sissies, we were prime targets for every splinter in the area, especially our hands.

My first line of treatment was my father. He was, after all, the one who always patched up our old tomcat, Tony. Tony's nocturnal avocations resulted in his coming home with substantial portions of his fur, skin, and ears missing. We went through many a bottle of A&P hydrogen peroxide on that cat, since vets were for rich kids' pets.

For wood splinters in our skin, Pa used the tried-and-true Army approach: sterilize a sewing needle (the bigger the better, it would seem) and unceremoniously dig the splinter out. This form of frontal attack worked, although of course, it also hurt. Once, however, I had a sliver way up under a fingernail. Even Dad backed away from that one. I was delighted when my folks sent me to our family doctor. There, I was certain, I would receive the adept and painless ministrations of a sympathetic healer.

Wrong.

The doctor sat me on his old-time, all-purpose, leather covered examination table, and painted my finger orange with lots of mercurochrome (23 percent mercury in a colorful solution). Then he turned to his little white cabinet of goodies and calmly produced a particularly large pair of black-handled office scissors. These are formidable-looking blades to see coming at your little fingertip.

Without a word, and without any anesthetic, the doctor began cutting away my fingernail. I was so surprised I could barely yell . . . for a moment, anyway. In a few agonizing minutes, he had removed over half the fingernail, and the splinter along with it. I decided that the mercurochrome's real role was to hide the color of the blood, which it very nearly did. But surely the pain of a forcibly removed fingernail is more suited to prisoner-of-war torture stories than to a doctor's office.

It was almost immediately afterward that I decided that not only could my father have done as well, I could have done as well myself. After all, we had a pair of ten-inch paper shears at home that were almost as big as the ones the doctor used.

The next time I had an under-the-finger sliver, I had the inspired idea to actively avoid the needle, or scissors, or battle ax, or whatever they might throw at me. I had some experience with "black drawing salve" (I think the brand of the day was Ichthamol). Black drawing salve is so-called because it is black (duh) and because it helps "draw" pus out of a wound or boil. I wondered if it would physically draw out a sliver of wood. So I applied a small glob of it, covered it with gauze, and waited.

The next morning, enough of the splinter was protruding from under my fingernail for me to simply grab it with tweezers and pull it out.

No pain. No blood. No skill needed.

How does this work? I have no idea. But I've seen it happen, time and time again.

Equipment list: black drawing salve (available at any discount drug store), your mother's eyebrow tweezers, and one Band-Aid.

Let's now up the ante somewhat and consider deep cuts and lacerations. How can we close them without stitches? With butterfly bandages, also available at any pharmacy or discount store.

Butterfly bandages look like doll-sized white paper bow ties. They are narrow in the middle, hence the name, and have a strong adhesive on the back. To use them properly, you first must staunch the flow of blood so you can see what you are doing, and ensure that they will stick. Pressure on or above the wound will usually do this. With a clean cloth or gauze, blot and dry the area as best you can. Do not use tissues or toilet paper, as these paper products will disintegrate when dampened and make a mess. Paper towels are okay. Remove the plastic adhesive-protecting strip from one side only of the bandage. This is easiest if you have an assistant help you. Then apply the bandage, like a bridge over troubled tissue, to hold the cut together. *The trick is to put a stretch into it.* To do so, you have to place the first side of the butterfly bandage further away from the cut than you'd think. When you pull it over, it will close the wound. Hold it, remove the adhesive-cover on the remaining side, and press it down to complete the maneuver. You can pre-remove the adhesive-covers from both sides in advance if it works better for you, but this is the way I do it.

Expect to make a schlock job of it the first time. Have at least half a dozen butterfly bandages on hand and do not worry if you have to scrap a few and try again. Keep the wound area as dry as possible, though, and you are likely to get it right on the first few tries.

Even if the first closure works well, I usually apply a second butterfly bandage. I do this even if the wound is a small one. I put the second one on at a slight angle to the first, to contact different skin and increase the likelihood of success. This results in an X shape that impresses children a great deal. Then I cover the X with a one-inch-wide Band-Aid. Or two. This helps lock the butterflies in place and, to a moderate extent, keeps them from getting wet. Wet bandages lose their stick and come off earlier. Better the outer ones than the butterflies, though, for it is easy to slap on a plain Band-Aid or two any time, any place. Ideally, you do not want to remove the butterfly closures for several days to a week, depending on the severity of the cut. This gives the skin a chance to knit together deep down as well as on the surface, and makes it unlikely that the wound will reopen.

On a long laceration, you can repeat the "bridging" process with a series of butterfly-bandage crosses. There is a limit to how far you can go with this, so get medical assistance whenever you need it.

Here's a hint: As the skin heals, it will tend to dry and "pull" and itch. Dropping some natural vitamin E onto the wound, simply squeezed from a pricked capsule, will help. Do not do this too early, for not only will the oil in vitamin E capsules completely ruin the bandage adhesive, but applied too soon, vitamin E's modest anticoagulant properties will delay surface clotting. Wait a few days to a week until you can see that the wound is solidly closed and you are ready to let the bandages come off anyway. As a side note, I might mention that if you want to spare your kids the pain of removing a bandage (slow or fast, it sure does hurt if there is hair under there), try this vitamin E technique. You will never hear an ouch again, for the bandages will easily come off on their own, and the kids will get the healing vitamin E benefits to boot.

In addition, healing is likely to be uncomplicated (no infection, scarring, or keloid formation) if you keep putting a tiny bit of vitamin E on the wound twice a day. Again, be sure the wound area is dry. Vitamin E oil and water don't mix. You can apply vitamin E to a conventional line of sutures, too. Overnight, it reduces soreness and swelling in and around the sutured area.

Bleeding is nature's way of cleaning a wound, so antiseptics and antibiotics are needed only rarely. If the wound is less than perfectly clean, I apply some iodine tincture to it, *but not right away,* because it hurts! Wait until you see slight redness after a couple of days. Iodine tincture is less disruptive of bandage adhesive than is vitamin E oil, and may be applied sooner, but sparingly. (You will need to carefully remove the outer covering of bandages to do this, of course, but you will want to see how the wound is coming anyway.) No need to remove the butterflies; just touch the iodine applicator to the exposed edge of the wound and it will be drawn in by itself. One or two applications is usually enough if you then follow up with the vitamin E treatment as mentioned above.

In summary:

1. Pressure to stop blood flow.

2. Dry the wound.

3. Butterfly bandage(s) applied with a stretch.

75

4. Cover with Band-Aid(s).

5. Add topical vitamin E after healing is well underway.

I may know how to do all this, but I confess that I still hate buying Band-Aids. This is because as a parent, I know all too well for whom I am buying them. I especially grimace when buying butterfly bandages. The only good thing about them is that they work as well or better than the alternative: stitches. I have only rarely had to use butterfly bandages on each of my children. Once my daughter fell in primary school and cut her chin. She had a Band-Aid on when she got off the bus. When we removed it, we saw that the cut was deep enough to expose yellow-orange fat. That is a deep cut. I very carefully applied a pair of butterfly bandages, which held the skin tightly together. After four or five days we started applying vitamin E to the site. Healing was so successful that you cannot find what surely would have been a scar had we gone the stitches route. When I had a chin laceration of my own some years before, I had stitches (not then knowing the butterfly technique). I have a scar to this day (which I hide nicely under my beard).

I have personally observed children getting stitched up in an emergency room. It is a scene to be avoided. In my daughter's case, it was. A laceration was effectively closed without needles, without the pain they necessarily cause, and without the stress of going to and waiting for assistance. I don't relish the task, but I'd prefer to be the one delivering care to my own kids. I think they greatly prefer it as well.

If it is a question of competence, then we must become competent, for even emergency room personnel might not be. "Many U.S. emergency rooms are staffed by doctors who were never taught how to treat a heart attack, resuscitate a child or treat bleeding," says the Rochester, New York *Democrat and Chronicle.* According to "Dr. L. Thompson Bowles, president of the National Board of Medical Examiners and chairmen of a group of 38 healthcare authorities who studied the issue . . . many [emergency room doctors] lack training and adequate experience in any aspect of primary health care."

Still, if you really need an ambulance, call one! Major traumatic injuries and some other situations absolutely demand medical technology. Even if the medical residents are not experienced, chances are the nurses and paramedics are. I submit, however, that we can reclaim a significantly larger part of our own health responsibility than most doctors would allow, and by simpler steps than most doctors would admit. I actually learned how to use the butterfly bandage from a friend over the phone, and by reading the directions on the package. It was time well spent to save my little girl from added pain and a facial scar.

Recommended Reading

Werner D. *Where There Is No Doctor: A Village Health Care Handbook.* Berkeley, CA: Hesperian Foundation, 1992. (Although allopathic in tone, this book remains a favorite of mine. It includes information on how to make your own butterfly bandages, how to suture a wound, how to set fractures, and pretty much anything else you can possibly think of.)

Before the FDA removed all tryptophan supplements from the market due to a temporary, and now corrected, industrial manufacturing error, millions of people had safely taken regular suppertime doses of this amino acid, usually 500–2,000 mg, to help them sleep. Inside you, tryptophan is broken down into anxiety-reducing, snooze-inducing niacin. Even more important, tryptophan is also made into serotonin, one of your body's most important neurotransmitters. Serotonin is responsible for feelings of well-being and mellowness. This is such a profound effect that Prozac, Paxil, and similar antidepressants artificially keep the body's own serotonin levels high. You can do the same thing naturally through diet. And no one can tell us that beans, peas, cheese, nuts, sunflower seeds, and good ol' wheat germ are toxic if you eat a lot of them!

Plenty of carbohydrates in your meals helps tryptophan get to where it does the most good: your brain. In order to cross the blood-brain barrier and get in, carbs are required. So cheese and crackers provides a better effect than the cheese standing alone. Cover your ears, animal friends, for I am also about to condone eating the occasional dead bird. Poultry, especially the dark meat, is a rich (yet very cheap) source of tryptophan. Add potatoes or stuffing, and you have the reason everybody is sprawled out and snoring up a storm after a typical Thanksgiving food orgy. But to be able to look your parakeet in the eye after the fourth Thursday in November, you can stay vegetarian and still get tanked up on tryptophan.

Consider that five servings of beans, a few portions of cheese or peanut butter, or several handfuls of cashews provide 1,000–2,000 mg of tryptophan, which will work as well as prescription antidepressants—but don't tell the drug companies. Some skeptics think that the pharmaceutical people already know, and that is why the FDA is keeping tryptophan supplements off the market. Here are two quotes in evidence:

"Pay careful attention to what is happening with dietary supplements in the legislative arena. . . . If these efforts are successful, there could be created a class of products to compete with approved drugs. The establishment of a separate regulatory category for supplements could undercut exclusivity rights enjoyed by the holders of approved drug applications."

FDA Deputy Commissioner for Policy David Adams, at the Drug Information Association Annual Meeting, July 12, 1993

"The task force considered many issues in its deliberations including to

ensure that the existence of dietary supplements on the market does not act as a disincentive for drug development."

FDA Dietary Task Force Report, released June 15, 1993

Remember that tryptophan is one of the ten essential amino acids you need to stay alive. It is by law added to liquid feedings for the elderly and all infant formulas. Yet tryptophan supplements remain illegal. You can legally buy L-5-hydroxytryptophan (5-HTP), a nonprescription tryptophan derivative, at health foods stores. 5-HTP is quite costly, however. The good news is that plenty of inexpensive vitamin C enables your body to convert dietary tryptophan into your own 5-HTP, and then on into serotonin.

So go, eat, and be happy!

Foods High in the Amino Acid L-Tryptophan

The source is the USDA, Amino Acid Content of Foods, and the **amounts are in milligrams per 100-gram (3.5-ounce) portion**, about the size of a deck of playing cards. That is not a large serving, and in a single meal, you might easily double or triple the figures listed here.

Beans

Lentils 215
Dried peas 250
Navy 200
Pinto 210
Red kidney 215
Soy 525

Nuts and Seeds

Brazil nuts 185
Cashews 470
Filberts 210
Peanuts 340
Peanut butter 330 (natural, not
    commercial)
Pumpkin seeds 560
Sesame seeds 330
Tahini (ground sesame seeds) 575
Sunflower seeds 340
Other nuts generally provide at least
    130 mg per small serving; usually
    more.

Grains

Wheat germ 265

Cheese

Cheddar 340
Parmesan 490
Swiss 375

Other cheeses tend to be lower in tryptophan, but are still very good sources.

Eggs 210

Poultry 250

(Note how vegetarian sources are as good as, and often much better than, flesh sources.)

Brewer's Yeast 700

Meats are generally regarded as a good source of tryptophan, organ meats supposedly being the highest. However, most meats are in the range of 160–260 mg/100 g, with organ meats ranging between 220 and 330. These figures certainly do not compel meat eating. They compel split pea, cheese, and cashew eating!

While in college, a friend of mine went to an expensive dermatologist because he had a slight rash. The specialist told him it was "dermatitis" and issued him a nifty cream to put on it. The visit cost my friend half a week's pay, and when he came to realize that "dermatitis" meant "itchy skin," he went ballistic. You might be able to save some space in your checkbook, and maybe even some time in the waiting room, with my very own "Ten Ways to Dodge Your Dermatologist."

1. Shampoo less often. If you are troubled by simple but annoying scalp conditions, this is really worth a try before you drop the big bucks on a doctor. A physician I go to for once-a-decade physicals prescribed not one but *two* antibiotics (one topical, one oral) for a chronic scalp irritation. He also recommended a very expensive shampoo and said to use it often. Nuts to that; the condition went away when I simply stopped shampooing every day and went to just once a week. Will this make your hair look all icky? Come on, now: do you shampoo your cat every day?

2. Use less soap. Not none, but less! I am not suggesting that you become the poster person for vagrancy; just use less of what everybody knows dries out skin. You use soaps and detergents to dissolve grease and oil when you wash your clothes and clean your dishes. We all know that soaps and detergents "cut grease." Right! They do the same to your skin, removing the natural oils that protect the skin—and the moisture and softness that no product can truly replace. A naturopath once told me that one should shower without soap, except for judicious application to personal areas that really need it.

3. Sunblock alone will not protect you from the sun. To avoid sunburn, wear a brimmed hat and loose, cool, comfy clothes instead. Simple, no? You'd be genuinely surprised just how many people still do not realize that the ozone layer is not what it was thirty years ago. More ultraviolet light (UV-B in particular) does in fact now reach us than was the case a generation or two ago. You can avoid practically all basal cell and squamous cell carcinoma, the two most common types of skin cancer, simply by putting on some clothes. I like a nice tan as much as the next person, but you simply have to use common sense here. Look: if you were diagnosed even with relatively easy-to-cut-out skin cancer, wouldn't you do just anything to be able to go back and prevent it? Even wear a hat and a shady shirt? Well, now is the time to start.

4. Switch to more natural perfumes, soaps, and deodorants. For this, you may need to stop by your local health food store. There really are many natural, gentle alternatives to the cheap, caustic, common cosmetic chemicals that irritate our skin! (Has the Pulitzer Prize in Alliteration been awarded yet?) I know two people who used to have numerous, small polyplike growths on their neck and underarms. These were no more than slightly unsightly, yet they were hardly an improvement to the basic birthday suit. In each case, they went away when the one person stopped using antiperspirant deodorants, and when the other stopped putting perfume directly on her skin. Read the label; even some "natural" deodorants are not that natural. However, most are a big improvement for a small cash difference.

5. Build skin health from the inside out. To have healthy skin, grow it. Your skin is an organ, like your lungs or heart, but a lot more visible, and a lot bigger, too. Your skin is, in fact, your body's largest organ. Feed your skin nutrients by eating more fiber, trying a vegetarian diet; and how about a few days of juice fasting? See for yourself if a healthy inside equals a healthy outside.

6. Chocolate: Stop eating it. It is no myth but a matter of observable fact that if you eat a good bit of chocolate, your skin will break out. If you cut out the chocolate, your skin will likely improve. Part of this is due to dietary fat; part is due to the chemical makeup of cocoa itself. Try and see. Hershey's common stock will do fine without your help.

7. Use less skin and hair glop. You'll save a pile of cash, and if you follow the suggestions above, you won't need all that stuff anyway. I remember a neat "Nancy" cartoon where she bathed and showered and dried her hair, then covered it with all the sprays, gels, mousses, and what have you. She looked in a mirror, realized how yucky her chemical hair was, and went back into the tub to wash it all off again. Okay, it wasn't the most hilarious cartoon I've ever seen (that, of course, would be the "Far Side" take on "the real reason dinosaurs became extinct"). But the point was made nonetheless.

8. Take your vitamins. Your skin really loves vitamin E (internally and externally), the B-complex vitamins, and assorted other nutrients that modern diets so often lack.

9. Eat more lecithin. Lecithin contains linoleic and linolenic acid, the absolutely essential fatty acids. As adult Americans try to reduce their fat intake (generally a good idea), no one has told them that they may thereby be creating a fatty acid deficiency. Since the government, the medical profession, and most dietitians just cannot own up to the necessity of food supplements, we had better consider them ourselves. The irritable-skin, dry-skin, broken-skin consequences of long-term linoleic and especially linolenic-acid deficiency are probably very common. I eliminated my own chronic dermatitis with just a few days supplementation of

three tablespoons of lecithin per day. A few tablespoons per week keeps it away. No dermatologist needed.

10. Reduce stress. (See my chapter "Stress Reduction" for specific suggestions.) A personal observation: I was under high stress at one job for about four years, and I noticed four things: (1) my hair got gray; (2) my hair started to come out in the comb; (3) when I started taking more vitamins, the hair stopped coming out; and (4) when I started doing the work I love, my hair stopped graying. In my opinion, I am less gray than I was in 1989. You can look at my untouched photo on my website, marvel at my toupee, guess my age, and mail me your answer. The winner will receive absolutely nothing.

I am kidding about the toupee; it's all mine.

One in every sixteen people has diabetes. Nearly three million Americans are on insulin. Many instances of blindness, amputations, and death (more than 160,000 annually) result from the circulatory complications of diabetes. Diabetes mellitus is a group of metabolic disorders in which the body does not produce sufficient insulin, the hormone used to metabolize glucose (blood sugar). When glucose isn't metabolized efficiently, blood sugar levels rise, and this leads to impaired energy, growth, and immune response. Over time, this can cause damage and eventual failure of many organs, including the heart, blood vessels, kidneys, nerves, and eyes.

Diabetes is divided into two prevalent forms. Type 1 diabetes, often called insulin-dependent or juvenile-onset, seems to be an autoimmune disease (where the body's own immune cells attack it) and is the most serious of the two. Type 2 diabetes, often called non-insulin-dependent or maturity-onset, generally occurs later in life, especially in overweight people, and is the result of poor diet and lifestyle habits: faced with a lifelong barrage of simple carbohydrates from sweets and refined starches, the pancreas eventually becomes exhausted and can no longer pump out enough insulin. Even many orthodox medical doctors agree with me that this one can be solved through diet and supplementation.

Five Musts for a Diabetic

1. **Eliminate Sugar.** No one would tell a child with a broken leg to jump off the garage roof. But perhaps we should not even let children *without* broken legs jump off garage roofs. Dieticians would never recommend that diabetics regularly eat lots of sweets. But really, no one should. The vast majority of us overconsume sugar to an alarming degree. Can this not only aggravate diabetes, but actually *cause* it? In the case of type 2, it is almost certainly so. And with type 1, the risk is there. There is no downside to avoiding sugar except, perhaps, putting your local dentist on unemployment. Avoid simple starches too, such as pasta, white rice, and white bread. These are quickly converted into sugars by the body. Instead, choose complex carbohydrates like whole wheat bread and brown rice. These are converted into sugars much more slowly.

2. **Avoid Milk.** Milk consumption in childhood can contribute to the development of type 1 diabetes. Certain proteins in milk resemble molecules on the beta cells of the pancreas that secrete insulin. In some cases, the immune system makes antibodies to the milk protein that mistakenly attack

and destroy the beta cells. Even so august an authority on children as the late Dr. Benjamin Spock changed his recommendations in his later years and discouraged giving children milk.

3. **Avoid Fluoride.** Even at only one tenth (0.4 ppm) of the U.S. government's maximum "safe" allowed level, fluoride is known to interfere with kidney function, and impaired ability to normally excrete fluoride has been found in people with diabetes. Fluoride accumulates in living systems—such as, say, your children. And it may accumulate especially fast in persons with nephrogenic diabetes, because of a polydipsia-polyurea syndrome that results in their increased intake, plus an abnormally high tendency to retain fluoride. Albert Burgstahler, Professor of Chemistry at the University of Kansas, says, "Children with nephrogenic diabetes insipidus or untreated pituitary diabetes have been found to develop severe dental fluorosis from drinking water containing only 1 or even 0.5 ppm fluoride" and that diabetics "are especially susceptible to the toxic effects of fluoride." Although fluoride is more poisonous even than lead, the Environmental Protection Agency allows over 250 times as much fluoride in your water as it allows lead in your water (4.0 ppm vs. 0.015 ppm). And the EPA's stated goal is to ultimately reduce lead levels to zero. No such luck with fluoride.

4. **Avoid Caffeine.** Caffeine is a drug, and can interfere with normal blood sugar levels. Caffeine magnifies the effects of the hormones glucagon and adrenaline, causing more sugar from the liver to be released into the blood stream. This means a raise in blood glucose levels. The more caffeine consumed, the more this is true.

5. **Question Immunization.** Be very cautious of vaccination. Medical historian Harris Coulter has observed that diabetes is ten times more common today in the United States than it was in the 1940s. The pertussis vaccine, in particular, has an impact on the insulin-producing centers in the pancreas. Overstimulation, and ultimate exhaustion, of these centers can lead to diabetes. The risk of type 1 diabetes may also be increased if the Hepatitis B vaccine is given to babies when they are six weeks old.

B-Complex Vitamins

One of the first nutrition zingers I ever read was Dr. Carlton Fredericks's comment in *Food Facts and Fallacies* that diabetics could be weaned off insulin with extremely high doses of B-complex vitamins. I am a conservative person and I have my sincere doubts if a type 1 diabetic could ever be entirely free of the need to take insulin. On the other hand, I have personally seen such diabetics require significantly less insulin when they take a 100 mg balanced B-complex tablet every two to three hours. The potential benefits are so great that I think diabetics should demand a suitably cautious therapeutic trial of megavitamin therapy *with insulin dosage adjustment made and supervised by their physicians.*

A daily dosage of 1,500 to 2,500 mg of niacin or niacinamide (one of the B-complex vitamins) may improve carbohydrate tolerance in diabetics. People with niacin deficiency may show hypersensitivity to insulin, with their blood sugar decreasing more readily than normal subjects after an injection of insulin. This means that niacin or niacinamide diminishes the requirements of insulin needed to keep the blood sugar of diabetics within normal limits. The dosage can be given in 500 mg amounts three to five times daily at first, then reduced as the blood sugar comes down.

A chiropractor in Pennsylvania wrote to me and said, "I recently had a pharmacist take one of my female diabetic patients off niacin (after an extremely successful course of therapy with niacin that eliminated years of insomnia) because he told her that it would mess up her blood sugar. I had another female diabetic patient who got some decent results with niacin for depression but was told by her pharmacist not to use it with diabetes. Yet I cannot seem to find anything to support *not* using niacin in diabetics."

That is simply because niacin works, and in doing so, creates a management issue. When megadoses of niacin lower the need for insulin, that is success, but an inconvenience (and perhaps an embarrassment) for the pharmophilic (drug-loving) health professional. But the main point must not be missed: A reduction in insulin requirement is good news for the patient. I would like to receive information about studies alleging evidence of any problems with niacin or niacinamide administration in diabetics. Please send it to drsaul@DoctorYourself.com.

Vitamin C

In his recent book *Vitamin C: Who Needs It?*, Emanuel Cheraskin says, "What do the experts tell us about a vitamin C connection in the control of sugar metabolism? We turned to five of the leading textbooks dealing with diabetes mellitus published during the last five years. Would you believe? There was not one word indicating any connection or a lack of correlation between ascorbic acid and carbohydrate metabolism? This is even more incomprehensible when one realizes that reviews of the literature as far back as 1940 showed that blood sugar can be predictably reduced with intravenous ascorbate." One case study suggests that for each gram (1,000 mg) of vitamin C taken by mouth, the amount of insulin required could be reduced by two units. Vitamin C may also help to keep capillaries from bursting, a major cause of diabetic complications, by increasing the elasticity of these smallest of blood vessels. Physicians investigated the effect of 600 mg per day of magnesium and 2,000 mg per day of vitamin C on a group of fifty-six non-insulin-dependent diabetics. The vitamin C improved control of blood sugar levels. It also lowered cholesterol and triglyceride levels, and reduced capillary fragility. Additionally, the magnesium lowered blood pressure in the subjects.

Magnesium

Magnesium is unusually important to the diabetic. Magnesium is needed to metabolize carbohydrates, and magnesium has a role in the production and utilization of insulin. Magnesium deficiency can increase insulin resistance, and therefore can worsen a type 2 diabetic's control of blood sugar. To compound the problem, high blood sugar increases urinary loss of magnesium in a person who already does not have enough of it. While there is disagreement as to how important this deficiency actually is for the diabetic, when has a long-term nutrient deficiency ultimately been proven to be beneficial? Taking a supplement providing at least the RDA of magnesium (about 400 mg) is, in my opinion, vital.

Exercise and Weight Control

Just do it! It helps tremendously. Suggestions on how are in my "Evading Exercise" chapter. Type 2 diabetes is clearly associated with overweight persons. Hint, hint.

Stress Reduction and Meditation

Diabetics (and most everyone else) will find that a wide variety of physical and mental benefits are among the advantages of regular, deep relaxation. The best relaxation techniques I have found are described in my chapter "Stress Reduction."

Chromium

The trace mineral chromium is found in skin, fat, muscle, brain tissue, and adrenal glands. There are only about 6 mg in you, but is that amount ever important! Absorption by way of your intestine is poor, and it is excreted in urine. Chromium is an essential component of Glucose Tolerance Factor (GTF). GTF helps insulin to work better by "bridging" it to cell membranes. Chromium as GTF improves glucose tolerance in diabetics whether they are children or adults.

Far and away the best food source of chromium is brewer's yeast. You can also use nutritional yeast, which is nutritionally similar and better tasting. Brewer's yeast is a byproduct of beer-making and tends to be a bit bitter. Nutritional yeast is primarily grown to be a food. Try nutritional yeast flakes on popcorn. It tastes so much like cheese that you may well like it. One Friday night, without telling what was in it, I sprung some of my stealthy, healthy ersatz "cheese popcorn" on some really finicky friends of mine. They happily munched away while trouncing me at euchre.

Aside from teaching them when to lead the left bower, one of the best things you can do is give your family a teaspoon or two of this stuff every day. In addition to chromium, it is a good source of B vitamins. Way too much, by the way, may cause temporary and harmless skin irritation in some especially sensitive people. If you start low and increase slow, this will probably not occur.

Other food sources of chromium include nuts, prunes, mushrooms, most whole grains, and many fermented foods, including beer and wine. Please remember the negative nutritional aspects of alcohol, and instead go for the yeast. If you simply must tip a few, at least try to select additive-free, organically grown beverages and use them in moderation.

If you are a teetotaler, and your interest in yeast is rapidly waning, the best supplements usually combine chromium with niacin, which seems to greatly enhance uptake. An example is chromium polynicotinate, which has been demonstrated to be especially well absorbed and retained. However, almost any chromium supplement will get decent results.

I would *always* supplement with 200–400 mcg of chromium daily if there is any hint of hypoglycemia (and that's most of us). In fact, I take that much every day. The RDA is 50–200 mcg daily. Even traditional diet textbooks admit that the conventional U.S. diet does not reliably supply even this amount. For the diabetic, chromium supplementation is essential . . . unless you are a *huge* fan of yeast.

Fiber

There is a well-established reduction of hyperglycemia in people who consume extra dietary fiber. This means a probable decrease in insulin requirement for type 1 diabetics, and even better news for type 2s. Generally, the more fiber eaten, the less medication needed. Try it and see how much better you feel. Soluble fiber, such as pectin (a thickener used to make jelly), may also help. It appears that even ever-delightful, over-the-counter Kaopectate has been used medically in the treatment of diabetes. Ugh. But the really good news is that fibers like pectin are found in the cell walls of all fruits and vegetables. Diabetics should eat a lot more vegetables.

Vitamin E

Persons with low vitamin-E levels have almost four times the risk of type 2 diabetes. Large quantities of vitamin E (1,800 IU daily) restored normal blood flow in the retina of the eyes of type 1 (insulin dependent) diabetics. The patients beginning the study with the worst readings were the ones who improved the most. Vitamin E may also reduce the risk for the development of retinopathy or nephropathy in diabetics. Vitamin E's strong protective influence suggests that damage by free-radicals may be a cause of these complications of the disease. Further information on vitamin E and diabetes can be found in the books of Evan and Wilfrid Shute, especially *Vitamin E for Ailing and Healthy Hearts*.

Vanadium

Some years ago, I had the pleasure of teaching clinical nutrition with Cornell University researcher Wes Canfield. Trace minerals are Dr. Canfield's special interest, and he believes that vanadate is very important in the prevention and treatment of diabetes, because of its ability to mimic insulin. Do not go belting down megadoses of vanadium just yet, however, as there are concerns about vanadium's potentially toxic side effects. A free search at the National Library of Medicine website (known as PubMed, www.nlm.nih.gov) will bring up some two hundred papers on vanadium.

Iatrogenic (Doctor-Caused) Diabetes

At least some instances of diabetes may be a major side effect of antibiotics and other common pharmaceuticals. Diabetes, usually thought to be largely of genetic or dietary origin, may be increasing so much in recent decades because of the proliferation in the use, and overuse, of medicines. To the extent that this is true, alternative measures need to be fully explored. I consider Melvyn Werbach's *Nutritional Influences on Illness,* and his more recent *Textbook of Nutritional Medicine,* to be must-reads. Werbach provides valuable summaries of research indicating the therapeutic value of various supplemental nutrients, and their specific dosages, for diabetics.

Recommended Reading

Balch JF and Balch PA. *Prescription for Nutritional Healing.* Garden City Park, NY: Avery Publishing, 1990.

Barnard RJ, et al. Response of non-insulin-dependent diabetic patients to an intensive program of diet and exercise. *Diabetes Care* 5 (1982): 370–74.

Bennett PH, et al. 1979. The role of obesity in the development of diabetes of the Pima Indians. In J. Vague and P.H. Vague, eds. Diabetes and Obesity. *Excerpta Medica,* Amsterdam.

Bruckert E, et al. Increased serum levels of Lipoprotein(a) in diabetes mellitus and their reduction with glycemic control. *JAMA* 263 (1990): 35–36.

Cheraskin E. *Vitamin C: Who Needs It?* New York: Arlington Press, 1993.

Cheraskin E, et al. Effect of caffeine versus placebo supplementation on blood glucose concentration. *Lancet* 1 (June 1967): 1299–1300.

Cheraskin E and Ringsdorf WM. Blood glucose levels after caffeine. *Lancet* 2 (September 1968): 21.

Classen JB. Childhood immunization and diabetes mellitus. *New Zealand Medical Journal* 195 (May 1996).

Corica F, et al. Effects of oral magnesium supplementation on plasma lipid concentrations in patients with non-insulin-dependent diabetes mellitus. *Magnes. Res.* 7 (1994): 43–46.

Coulter H. "Childhood Vaccinations and Juvenile-Onset (Type-1) Diabetes." Testimony before the Congress of the United States, House of Representatives, Committee on Appropriations, Subcommittee on Labor, Health and Human Services, Education, and Related Agencies, April 16, 1997.

Cunningham JJ, Mearkle PL, and Brown RG. Vitamin C: an aldose reductase inhibitor that normalizes erythrocyte sorbitol in insulin-dependent diabetes mellitus. *J Am Coll Nutr* 13 (August 1994): 344–45.

Dental fluorosis associated with hereditary diabetes insipidus. *Oral Surgery* 40 (1975): 736–41.

Dice JF and Daniel CW. The hypoglycemic effect of ascorbic acid in a juvenile-onset diabetic. *International Research Communications System* 1 (1973): 41.

Eriksson J and Kohvakka A. Magnesium and ascorbic acid supplementation in diabetes mellitus. *Annals of Nutrition and Metabolism* 39 (July/Aug 1995): 217–23.

Fredericks C and Bailey H. *Food Facts and Fallacies.* NY: Arco, 1995.

Garrison RH and Somer E. *The Nutrition Desk Reference.* New Canaan, CT: Keats, 1990 216–22.

Hoffer A. *Vitamin B-3 (Niacin) Update; New Roles For a Key Nutrient in Diabetes, Cancer, Heart Disease and Other Major Health Problems.* New Canaan, CT: Keats Publishing,1990.

Hoffer A and Walker M. *Orthomolecular Nutrition.* New Canaan, CT: Keats Publishing, 1978, 14, 21–26, and 100–101.

Junco LI, et al. "Renal Failure and Fluorosis," Fluorine and Dental Health. *JAMA* 222 (1972): 783–85.

Kapeghian JC, et al. The effects of glucose on ascorbic acid uptake in heart, endothelial cells: Possible pathogenesis of diabetic angiopathies. *Life Sci* 34 (1984): 577.

Mather HM, et al. Hypomagnesemia in diabetes. *Clinical and Chemical Acta* 95 (1979): 235–42.

McNair P, et al. Hypomagnesemia, a risk factor in diabetic retinopathy. *Diabetes* 27 (1978): 1075–77.

Pfleger R and Scholl F. Diabetes und vitamin C. *Wiener Archiv für Innere Medizin* 31(1937): 219–30.

Salonen JT, et al. Increased risk of non-insulin dependent diabetes mellitus at low plasma vitamin E concentrations: a four year follow-up study in men. *BMJ* 311 (October 1995): 1124–27.

Setyaadmadja ATSH, Cheraskin E, and Ringsdorf WM. Ascorbic acid and carbohydrate metabolism: II. Effect of supervised sucrose drinks upon two-hour postprandial blood glucose in terms of vitamin C state. *Lancet* 87 (January 1967): 18–21.

Sinclair AJ, et al. Low plasma ascorbate levels in patients with type 2 diabetes mellitus consuming adequate dietary vitamin C. *Diabet Med* 11 (November 1994): 893–98.

Snowdon DA and Phillips RL. Does a vegetarian diet reduce the occurrence of diabetes? *Am J Public Health* 75 (1985): 507–12.

Som S, et al. Ascorbic acid metabolism in diabetes mellitus. *Metabolism* 30 (1981): 572–77.

Stone I. *The Healing Factor: Vitamin C Against Disease.* New York: Grosset & Dunlap, 1972, 146–51.

Timimi FK, et al. Vitamin C improves endothelium-dependent vasodilation in patients with insulin-dependent diabetes mellitus. *J Am Coll Cardiol* 31 (March 1998): 552–57.

Toxicological Profile for Fluorides, Hydrogen Fluoride, and Fluorine (F). Agency for Toxic Substances and Disease Registry, U.S. Dept. of Health and Human Services, April 1993, 112.

Werbach M. *Nutritional Influences on Illness.* New Canaan, CT: Keats Publishing, 1988.

Werbach M. *Textbook of Nutritional Medicine.* With Jeffrey Moss. Tarzana, CA: Third Line Press, 1999.

Williams SR. *Nutrition and Diet Therapy,* 6th edition, chapter 19. St. Louis, MO: Mosby, 1989.

Ask any of the 5 million women who have it, and they will tell you just how miserable endometriosis can be. In this chronic disease, tissue (endometrium) that you would expect inside the uterus ends up outside of it, often throughout the pelvic cavity. The monthly menstrual cycle aggravates the problem with (among other things) internal bleeding, inflammation, and considerable pain and discomfort.

Selenium

In cattle, endometriosis can be due to selenium deficiency. Since your cow can't give you any milk without having a baby first, dairymen well know to supplement all cows' feed with selenium. This is usually accomplished with a multimineral tablet the size of a microwave oven. Okay, it's a mineral-fortified salt block (after all, salt *is* a mineral) that cows can lick any time they want.

Human females should do it as well, but they don't.

We go out of our way to supply selenium to cattle, particularly in geographical regions that have selenium-poor soil. Farmers simply must have healthy, fertile, happily pregnant, uncomplicated-delivering Bossys by the herd. It's economics: farmers cannot afford otherwise; a herd with endometriosis would be bankruptcy on the hoof.

Women with endometriosis, on the other hand, mean an economic windfall for doctors, nurses, support staff, surgeons, hospitals, administrators, HMOs, insurance companies, pharmaceutical manufacturers, drug salespeople, and lots of others dependent on unwell people.

The secret to endometriosis is to see it for what it is: an end result of malnutrition. Farmers see this. Physicians do not. Cows are raw-food vegetarians who obtain their minerals from grains, leafy greens, and smart dairymen who provide mineral supplements preventively. Physicians and their ilk try to treat endometriosis (1) after it has occurred, and (2) with drugs.

Endometriosis is not due to a drug deficiency. It may be due to a selenium deficiency. Selenium is probably important in stopping endometriosis because this trace mineral works so closely with vitamin E. Vitamin E has been known to ensure that animals have healthy uterine linings since the 1930s. The research trail on this is as long as your arm. Therefore, supplementing the diet of a human female with natural vitamin E, 400–1,000 IU daily, plus 100–200 mcg selenium, is a good move.

Folate (Folic Acid)

I suspect folate deficiency as a cause of endometriosis. To some extent I base this opinion, once again, on cows. And I repeat that cows are vegetarians. Raw-food vegetarians.

Folate is named after the dark green leafy vegetables it was first extracted from. "Folium" is Latin for leaf. Folic acid contains three parts: pteroic acid, glutamic acid, and para-aminobenzoic acid (PABA). Folate is an important coenzyme in your body, helping to move carbon units around, and is necessary for synthesis of the nitrogen-containing purines and pyrimidines essential for the synthesis of nucleotides, which make up your RNA and DNA. Folate is also necessary for making the heme (the iron-containing, nonprotein part of hemoglobin) in your red blood cells.

Too little folate causes megoblastic anemia (that's large, immature red blood cells that can't carry oxygen well). This is especially important during growth situations, such as pregnancy, infancy, and childhood.

Cows get plenty of folate because they eat plenty of foliage (leafy green stuff, like grass). They are also blissfully free from a silent folate-stealer: the birth control pill. Oral contraceptives dramatically increase (at least double) the need for folic acid in women. And disease in general increases need for folic acid.

Adolescents in particular are likely to have insufficient folic acid intake. Why? Because food sources of folate are often quite unpopular. They are:

1. leafy green vegetables (Teens *love* these. Not.)

2. organ meats ("Awesome!")

3. asparagus ("McSparagus! My favorite fast food!")

During the growth period when they need it most, teenagers are likely not getting adequate dietary folic acid. Female teenagers reaching menarche (the beginning of menstruation) are therefore malnourished. Folate undernutrition is probably a factor in endometriosis.

Other nutrients recommended to help combat endometriosis include vitamin C in quantity, the vitamin B complex, essential fatty acids (found in lecithin or primrose oil), iron, iodine, calcium, and magnesium. Dietary supplementation makes sense to try.

Raspberry leaves are rich in magnesium and have a long tradition of uterine usefulness. I have seen raspberry-leaf tea reduce pregnancy problems and delivery times in humans. We fed piles of raspberry leaves to our rabbit, who rewarded us with ten young practically while our backs were turned. That is a large litter even for a rabbit.

Pregnancy and endometriosis are not in a cart-and-horse relationship: it is not known for certain which one influences the other. But I think the less sure we are, the more we should look to nature for our examples. What is good for heifers is good for humans. I vote for a bovine diet, plus supplements.

Recommended Reading

Balch J and Balch P. *Prescription for Nutritional Healing.* Garden City Park, NY: Avery, 1990.

Williams S. *Nutrition and Diet Therapy,* 6th edition. St. Louis, MO: Mosby, 1989.

Sarah and her fiancé Richard wanted to have children as soon as they were married. Sarah had just been diagnosed with epilepsy, however, and was taking phenobarbital as therapy. She and Richard read up on the drug, and now knew, as did their doctor, that a pregnancy on barbiturates was not ideal.

"So we want to look into other options," Sarah said to me in the office. "Could vitamins replace the drug?"

"I'm not sure," I said. "My mother has been medicated for grand mal epilepsy for fifty years now and it's a real long shot to think that a nutrient could be enough. Still, Sarah, you have the advantage of being young. There is evidence that epilepsy in teenagers can be connected with magnesium deficiency. You've had blood tests done?"

"Oh, yes," she said. "Tons of them, and here's the latest." She handed me a copy. No one had even looked for serum magnesium. I told Sarah to ask her doctor to check next time. So they did. Sarah's serum magnesium levels were so low as to be actually unmeasurable.

"The doctor was a bit surprised at that," Sarah said the next time we talked. "So now what?"

"Let's try a large quantity of magnesium, starting with a supplement of 800 mg per day. That's just over twice the RDA, so it is not completely unreasonable. Then you can gradually work up from there if need be. You'll know if you are taking too much: the biggest side effect of too much magnesium is diarrhea. You've heard of milk of magnesia?"

"The laxative, sure."

"That is a magnesium preparation. Your supplement will be better absorbed, though. Especially if you take the right form, take it often, and really need it. Then your body will soak it up like a sponge. Try magnesium citrate, or magnesium gluconate. Divide your daily intake over four or more doses, at least. Then let's see what we get."

A few weeks later, we met again. Sarah had new bloodwork results in hand. Her magnesium level was just barely measurable, and she was taking 1,200 mg a day.

"Wow! Where's it all going?" Sarah asked. "I've had no loose bowels at all."

"Your body is evidently using it. This suggests a long-standing deficiency on your part. Most young men and nearly all young women do not eat even the RDA of magnesium. But this is beyond that. You have a special need for this mineral. The tests confirm that."

"But shouldn't the blood levels be going up more?" Sarah asked.

"You'd think so, but not necessarily. You are more than your blood, important though blood certainly is. Serum tests fail to indicate how much of this or that is actually inside your body's cells. There are, after all, some 40 trillion of them. Magnesium is involved in hundreds of chemical reactions throughout your body. It is needed everywhere and always. Oddly enough, the cells can be critically low in magnesium and some of the mineral will often still show up in the serum. In your case, it's more the other way around. Now that you are supplementing with magnesium, your cells must be getting it, and there's not much left in the blood that transports it. There are a lot of tanker trucks on your highways, but they're empty. The cargo is delivered and now the fuel is in every home."

"So it looks like I need more magnesium than most people," said Sarah. "If I do take lots of it, will I need less of the drug?"

"That's the idea. Do you want to run it by your doctor? Ask him if he'd consider gradually decreasing your dose of phenobarbital down to the minimum that keeps you symptom-free."

She did, and he did. Sarah ended up on the lowest possible dose of the drug and a very high dose of magnesium. This was not a landslide victory for nutrition, but this book is about real solutions, not rhetoric: nutrition does not have to be an all-or-nothing proposition. Its greatest potential may be in maintaining optimally nourished bodies that then will thrive on vastly reduced medication. What are the long-term consequences of millions of Americans taking less of each of their many drugs? Healthier people, greater safety, and massive savings. Only the pharmaceutical companies could possibly object.

They do, of course. And, they heavily influence practicing physicians. When was the last time you saw a calendar, pen, ad, or prescription pad in your doctor's hand touting the benefits of magnesium?

Keep looking. It will be in some quack's office, no doubt.

Or not. L. B. Barnett, M.D., was onto this forty-five years ago. He published "Clinical Studies of Magnesium Deficiency in Epilepsy" in *Clinical Physiology* in 1959. Wonder why nobody listened?

If I assert that you can probably accomplish more with bean sprouts than with laser surgery, you'll call me some kind of a quack, which, to most people, I am.

Terri certainly thought I was. Terri was going blind, and she was miserable. She had a somewhat rare condition where her eyesight was tunneling. That is, Terri's peripheral vision was fading fast. She was still in her thirties. "This has just gotten worse and worse," she told me. "My sight is limited to what is right in front of me, and that's not very clear either. I can't drive. I can hardly even read any more."

"What has your ophthalmologist told you?" I asked.

"That there is nothing he can do, except monitor how much vision I've lost," she said. "A lot of good that does me."

"Surgery? Medications?"

"He said none are any help with what I've got," she said, her mouth firmly set. "I don't suppose you have any great ideas?"

I did have an idea or two, but she wasn't going to like them. "Naturopaths have accumulated decades of evidence about the food enzymes in uncooked foods, especially sprouted beans and sprouted grains. Cooking temperatures as low as 130 degrees Fahrenheit destroy these enzymes, which are essential to keeping us youthful and healthy."

"That sounds pretty cutesy," said Ms. Congeniality.

"It does to me, too. But I cannot discount the possibility, since you have been offered nothing else, that this research might apply to you. You could try a 90 percent raw food, mostly sprouts, diet for a few months."

"A few months?"

"At least. What I have read emphasizes that while nature heals, it takes time. The nature-cure authorities generally agree that it took years for our body to develop an affliction, and it will take us months to get out of it."

"If it works at all," said Terri.

"Yes, if it works at all."

There was a long silence. Counseling training, plus years of teaching, had taught me when to shut up and wait for a student to elaborate on their initial answer. "I'll try it," she finally said, "but this had better be worth it. How much of this stuff do I have to eat?"

Familiar question to a quack who raised two kids on sprouts. My children will readily tell you that I gave them sprouts for breakfast, carrot-zucchini juice for lunch, and borscht for supper. While that is true, it is not the complete story. My policy was "Eat this good-for-you item first, and then you can have what you want, within reason." My kids had plenty of ice cream, brownies, cookies, health-food-store candies, and other goodies on a regular basis. I get a lot of heat from purists who think I was a sell-out. But I got far more heat from their mother and my in-laws about the weird health foods I fed those "poor children." Compromise is a fact of life. If you hold too firmly to your principles, you risk them being discarded lock, stock, and barrel. But I felt that, in Terri's case, she would need to bite the nutritional bullet.

"You'll need to eat at least two jars full of sprouts a day," I told Terri. "By jars, I mean mayonnaise-sized or mason jars, about a quart and a half each. By sprouts, I mean a variety of alfalfa, wheat, lentil, radish, cabbage, clover, and mung bean. You can grow your sprouts yourself. That will save a lot of money, and they will be fresher and better for you."

"Ugh," replied Terri.

"Actually, sprouts taste better than you think. A lot of salad bars have alfalfa sprouts. Radish sprouts taste exactly like radishes. Mung bean sprouts are used in Chinese food. Try different varieties and mixtures. Any health food store or food co-op will have the seeds. Soak them overnight, and then rinse and drain them twice a day. Start two or three jars a day, and harvest and eat them in rotation as they mature. That's it."

"Eat them how?" asked the impatient patient.

"Raw, except perhaps for mung sprouts. Build your salads on a base of sprouts instead of lettuce. Eat sprouts in a sandwich instead of lettuce. Top sprout salads with tomatoes, cucumber, broccoli, cashew nuts, onion, salad dressing, anything."

"Dressing?" said Terri, with a glimmer of optimism. "I can have dressing on them? I thought dressing was full of salt and fat."

"Put anything you want on your sprouts to make them taste good. You want this to be as enjoyable as possible. I'll look the other way on whatever it takes to get you to consume as great a volume of sprouts a day as you can. The value of the sprouts far outweighs any drawback of the dressing. You can always make your own, if you really want to do it right. It really isn't that hard to eat a lot of sprouts. You can take nearly a jarful and press them down between two pieces of bread and make a sproutwich."

Silence.

"You'll also want to have fresh vegetable juices daily for all the carotenes, lots of vitamin B-complex, vitamin C and vitamin E, a good multivitamin, extra zinc, and a little selenium." We went over the recommended dosages. I suggested 600–1,200 IU daily of vitamin E, 100 mg per day of zinc, vitamin C to bowel tolerance (see my vitamin C chapter), and a B-complex pill with each meal. "Don't take too much selenium; 400 mcg a day is the maximum, and half that will probably be sufficient. The other nutrients have a safety record a mile long. The vegetable juice is better than beta-carotene supplements. Yes, it contains a great deal of beta-carotene, but it also contains dozens of other carotenes, not just the beta form. Even a single carrot a day reduces a person's risk of macular degeneration by 40 percent."

"I'll be taking pills all day," Terri grumbled.

"All these nutrients have an especially vital role in the health of the eye. Carotenes, C, E, zinc, and selenium are all involved with the antioxidant cycle. Macular degeneration, cataracts, and diabetic retinopathy are distantly related conditions that have responded to these nutrients."

Off she went, certainly no more miserable than when she came in, but that isn't saying much. Terri fundamentally questioned what she was doing, but driven by a lack of options, with that bare desperation that can work wonders, she did it. Kicking and screaming, perhaps, but she did it.

One phone conversation five weeks later, I dared ask her if she was noticing anything good happening.

"No," she said. "I went to the eye doctor this week, and he said there was no change."

"But isn't that actually a good sign, Terri? Every other visit, didn't he say that your vision was diminishing?"

"Well, yeah, he did."

"Then 'no worse' is an early sign of real progress," I said.

"Maybe. I hate eating sprouts."

"Look, Terri, I give you permission to hate my guts if it will keep you on the wagon and help you see."

She asked if she could have some rye bread. She asked if the bread could be toasted. She wanted some yogurt. (I said yes to all three.) The other day she had a piece of chicken. It was a dietetic confessional each time she called. And she called often.

Another month later, she had been to the ophthalmologist again. "He looked and said things were a bit better. He tested my vision and confirmed it. He asked what I was doing, and I told him you'd call him and explain it."

So I did, hoping for the best. The ophthalmologist was actually very interested. He noted some of my references, expressed his pleasure that Terri was improving with a condition that never improved, and said whatever she was doing, she shouldn't change it a bit. End of conversation.

Months went by, and Terri's eyesight got better and better. In the end, two near miracles happened: Terri's eyesight was restored nearly 100 percent, and she thanked me for what I'd made her do.

I will never forget what a wonderful feeling it was to have been the educational and motivational link that stopped Terri from going blind. It does not matter how a person gets their sight back. By divine healing from above, or by sprouted seeds of the earth; whatever works and restores something as precious as eyesight must be taken as genuine, and good.

Iget a lot of questions about natural birth control, usually about options to drug or barrier methods of contraception. Can a safe, natural alternative really cost nothing and be more than 99 percent effective? As a former school sex-education coordinator and author of a master's thesis on the subject, I will now offer a few fertile thoughts.

Even if it is granted that birth control education should begin very early, and that fertility awareness is a desirable inclusion, some objections may remain. One such objection is that there is no reliable indicator of fertility. This erroneous belief is widely held. A woman's cervical mucus secretion is a most reliable indicator of fertility. Using this fact to prevent conception is the basis for the Billings Method of birth control.

The Billings Method is named after Drs. John and Evelyn Billings of Melbourne, Australia, who first developed, tested, and promoted this natural birth control method in the 1950s. It is also known as the Ovulation Method or the Mucus Method. It is not the Rhythm Method. In fact, the reason the Billings began their investigation of natural birth control in the first place is because the Rhythm Method is not reliable.

Natural birth control often conjures up images of ineffectiveness and Catholicism. This is unfortunate. Even the Rhythm Method, when carefully employed, may be 80 percent effective in preventing pregnancy. But since that failure rate is still far too high, there have been attempts to improve on it. The Temperature Method is one of the best-known refinements on rhythm. It is based on an observed temperature rise at the time of a woman's ovulation each month. Three days after this temperature rise, she is infertile until at least the next menstrual period. While temperature indicates ovulation, it fails to predict it. Intercourse before the thermal shift, then, again becomes a matter of rhythm-style calendar estimation. Another drawback is identifying the temperature rise. A significant temperature rise may be as low as 0.1 degree centigrade, making this otherwise reliable method difficult to use.

The Billings Method simplifies natural birth control greatly. Its refinements are that it requires no equipment (no thermometer, no calendar), no guesswork, and that it will predict ovulation. It is simple enough that, according to the Billings, "Experience has shown that an overwhelming majority of women, probably nine out of ten, can immediately interpret their own mucus system. . . . The remainder can also be taught to do so."

The Billings Method is a one-step reading of a woman's cervical mucus, performed by the woman herself in a moment and without internal examination. Every day, she gently wipes her labia with clean, dry, white toilet paper.

She looks at the paper to see if there is any mucus on it. If there is, she is likely to be fertile. If the mucus is wet and slippery, and can be easily stretched, then she is very fertile. If the paper stays dry, she is likely to be infertile that day. On the day of the most wet, slippery, clear mucus, she is most fertile of all. This day is called the peak day, and is the very day she ovulates. She will also feel wettest on this day. She remains fertile for three days after the peak.

It does not matter how old the woman is, nor does it matter how long her menstrual cycles are. Unlike the Rhythm Method, there is no need for regular menstrual cycles. There is no need to fit into a normal, clockwork 28-day model. If a woman has short menstrual cycles, she will ovulate early. If they are long, she will ovulate late. The mucus is there at ovulation, regardless. If she misses a period, there will simply have been no ovulation, and therefore no fertile, wet mucus that cycle. A woman does not even have to know how to read and write to use the Billings Method effectively. Trials in the South Pacific nation of Tonga between 1970 and 1972 showed high levels of acceptance and success with the Billings Method.

Abnormal temperature, such as a low fever, will interfere with the temperature method of birth control. It will not obstruct accurate readings with the Billings Method, however. Abnormal vaginal discharges, also, do not prevent a woman from recognizing her state of fertility. Given the knowledge, any woman can use the Billings Method for her entire reproductive lifetime without financial cost. And, obviously, unlike medical methods of birth control, there are no harmful side effects with the Billings Method.

Few physicians and nurses know of the ovulation method's effectiveness, and fewer still teach it. Pity, since, according to John Billings, "The combined biological failure rate and user failure rate of the ovulation method in Tonga was 0.69 percent." This is very low indeed, since some experts place the birth control pill failure rate at 1.2 percent. Planned Parenthood says that excellent use of natural birth control can be up to 99 percent effective.

A nurse-midwife taught my wife and I the Billings Method in half an hour. It took another few hours to read their book, *The Ovulation Method.* We subsequently used the Billings Method for fifteen years and the method, properly used, never resulted in an unplanned pregnancy.

Caution: As with any birth control method, the Billings Method should be learned from an experienced instructor. Even more important, it obviously provides no protection whatsoever from sexually transmitted diseases. This is one of the most important reasons why it is appropriate only for strictly monogamous, long-term relationships.

By the way, you can use the method backward to assist conception, since the days on which a woman is ovulating are when she is most fertile.

Male Fertility

And now to enrage the gynecologists, fertility specialists, and dietitians.

If you want to conceive, try having the man take megadoses of vitamin C for a few weeks. At least 6,000 mg a day, and as much as 20,000 mg a day, guarantees a mighty high sperm production. Divide the dose throughout the day for maximum effect. More sperm, stronger sperm, and better-swimming sperm all occurred, at even lower daily C doses, in a University of Texas study. Take more C and you'll make vast quantities of super sperm. You think this won't work? Have I shown you pictures of all my kids?

Here's more: zinc and plenty of it helps the prostate and increases seminal fluid production. There is scientific literature a mile long about zinc and male fertility. About five to ten times the RDA will do it: 50–100 mg of zinc daily. For best absorption and best results, divide the dose into two, or better yet, four doses. Zinc gluconate is well absorbed, and zinc monomethionine better still. These are available at any health food store without a prescription. Take zinc supplements with food.

A lot of wussy nutritionists will tell you that such levels of zinc are harmful. Truth is, most men don't even get the puny RDA of zinc, set laughingly at 10–12 mg. Zinc lozenges for the common cold are many times higher than this. Up to 550 mg of zinc have been safely given daily for a few weeks.

Continued high doses of zinc can produce a copper deficiency, which can lead to anemia. This is very easy to compensate for. To begin with, most Americans have copper water pipes in their homes. Drink a glass or two of the first cold water out of the tap every morning and you'll get copper. Second, eat more raisins, whole grains, leafy green vegetables, and other copper-high foods. Third, take a multivitamin (as you should be doing anyway) with copper in it. Finally, do what fertile folks in India have been doing for thousands of years. Buy a copper metal cup, fill it with cold water at bedtime, and drink it first thing the next morning. Make zinc, copper, and vitamin C part of your routine, and start knitting booties.

I have worked with supposedly infertile people who have tried "everything" to conceive a child. Nutrition, especially the vitamin C part, is not even mentioned in any fertility textbook I've ever seen. I've received some nice postcards from couples who have taken an odd idea or two of mine and gotten pregnant within a month. It is a wonderful feeling to have helped them bring a soul into the world.

Recommended Reading

Billings J. Cervical mucus: the biological marker of fertility and infertility. *International Journal of Fertility* 26 (1981): 182–195.

Billings J. Ovulation method of family planning. *The Lancet* 2 (1972): 1193–94.

Billings J. *The Ovulation Method*. Collegeville, MN: Liturgical Press, 1978.

Billings J. In *Sex and Pregnancy in Adolescence,* Zelnik M, Kantner J, and Ford K, ed. Beverly Hills, CA: Sage, 1973, 164–70.

Billings J and Billings E. Teaching the safe period based on the mucus symptom. *Linacre Quarterly* 41 (1974): 41–51.

Clift AF. Observations on certain rheological properties of human cervical secretion. *Proceedings of the Royal Society of Medicine* 39 (1945): 1–9.

Doring GK. "Detection of Ovulation by the Basal Body Temperature Method" in *Sex and Pregnancy in Adolescence* by Zelnik M, Kantner J, and Ford K, ed. Beverly Hills, CA: Sage, 1973.

Klaus H. Valuing the precreative capacity: a new approach to teens. *International Review of Natural Family Planning* 8 (1984): 206–13.

Klaus H, et al. Fertility awareness—natural family planning for adolescents and their families: Report of multisite pilot project. *International Journal of Adolescent Medicine and Health* 3 (1987): 101–19.

Klaus H, Labbok M, and Barker D. Characteristics of ovulation method acceptors: a cross-cultural assessment. *Studies in Family Planning* 19 (1988): 299–304.

National Directory of Billings Ovulation Method Teachers. Washington, D.C.: Natural Family Planning Center of Washington, D.C., 1988.

"Teen STAR program." [pamphlet] Bethesda, MD: Natural Family Planning Center of Washington, D.C., 1986.

Weissman MC, et al. A trial of the ovulation method of family planning in Tonga. *The Lancet* 2 (1972): 813–16.

"What's the best method of birth control for me?" Rochester, NY: Planned Parenthood of Rochester and the Genesee Valley, 1986.

What natural approaches might help fibromyalgia?
Radical decapitation, perhaps?

After all, how many times have folks been told that their nagging pain and intense soreness are all in their heads? As late as 1982, "fibromyalgia" was not even an entry in the doctor's standard clinical reference book, the *Merck Manual.* You can find "myalgia," though, which is described as simple muscular pain. A predictable medical recommendation promptly follows: take an aspirin!

The most effective therapy I know for fibromyalgia is saturation of vitamin C along with the use of calcium/magnesium supplements. This seems too easy for a problem that so many have really suffered from, I know. But just ask anyone with fibromyalgia this question: Have you tried it yet? If they still have the condition, I'll bet they haven't tried it. Large doses of vitamin C seem to have exceptional anti-inflammatory properties. Saturation of vitamin C is easily reached through frequent oral doses, and is fully described in the chapter "Vitamin C Megadose Therapy."

Media scare-stories to the contrary, the safety and the effectiveness of large amounts of vitamin C are well established. Vitamin C is *far* safer than aspirin. Do not be put off by the very thing that can help the most until you have looked into it for yourself.

Calcium and magnesium supplementation, even at rather low RDA levels (about 1,000 mg calcium and 400 mg magnesium daily, in divided doses), can make a big difference in muscle health and happiness. A deficiency of either mineral can cause muscle pain and muscle problems. Dietary deficiency is the rule, rather than the exception, with both of these important minerals.

Gentle to moderate exercise can often help, too. Start light and gradually work up. Yoga stretches and walking are two good choices. Heavy weight-bearing workouts may set you back, so take it easy.

Want one more secret weapon? Vegetable juicing! I never feel so good, so energetic, so un-sore (is that a word?) as when I juice bigtime. Again, if you have not tried this utterly nontoxic approach to better health, why not? See my chapter "Juicing" for more information.

Or, you can just get some nice hydrocortisone injections to go along with the aspirin.

Todd was two, nearly. His mother brought him in to discuss options, if any, to scheduled surgery for his anal fistula. Todd had had a boil right next to his anus, and it had been lanced by a doctor. As is often the case, the drainage of pus left a pocket, which opened into a crevice. Nice, huh?

I first learned about this standard course of events from a surgical resident as he lanced the ugliest boil I could ever imagine. It was an inch long, half an inch wide, and immediately above the anus of a man, lying face down on an examining table, whose legs and butt were the only things protruding from under a white gown. At the time, I was a student observing at the emergency and outpatient surgical section of a local hospital. I rotated among several house staff, who showed me the ropes, among other things. The resident put a beige plastic cup between the guy's legs as he lay there, spread-eagled. A few jabs of lidocaine, and then a single stab with the knife. A fountain of white pus gushed from the incision. It was several teaspoons, easily. Gross. The resident matter-of-factly said that the man would probably develop a fistula there, which would need to be dealt with when it happened.

My mind came back to the present, where Todd was wandering around my office, hauling a few toys out of the box I kept handy for bored kids. He looked over at his mother, smiling. Had Todd known what was in store for him, he wouldn't have smiled at all. He was to travel to Boston for surgery at a specially selected hospital that allowed parents to stay overnight with their children. In the meantime, however, his mother asked if there were any alternatives to the surgical repair itself.

"I doubt it," I said. "It's asking a lot of a vitamin to close up a fistula without suturing it."

"What about the pus that keeps oozing out?" the mother asked. "This has been going on almost daily since the boil was drained."

"Perhaps there is something that might help that," I said. "You could try a homeopathic remedy called silicea. It's a harmless, over-the-counter preparation that has been used for pus-producing conditions for over a century. It's actually a microdilution of the main mineral in common sand, silica."

"A mineral? That sounds safe enough. Where would I buy it?" she asked.

"Any health food store. I usually used the 6X potency with my kids. The "X" is like the Roman numeral; it stands for ten. The "6" means it has been diluted six successive times. That's less than one part per million."

"Your kids had fistulas, too?" asked Todd's mom.

"No, but they've had a boil once or twice elsewhere, and so have I," I added. "The silicea cleared it up in a day or two. Never had any medicine or needed lancing. As long as you're waiting for the surgery anyway, it's worth trying it in the meantime."

Because of the number of times I'd seen silicea work, I was actually pretty confident that it would stop the pus problem. And, because of what I'd seen of fistulas, that's all I expected.

A joyful woman was on the phone a week later. "The fistula is gone!" said Todd's mother. "Not only did it stop the pus, the fistula closed up! Could the silicea have done all that?"

"Can't argue with success," I said. "Take Todd into his pediatrician and have her take a look."

"Already did that!" said the mom. "We canceled the surgery!"

Calls like that make my day. Calls like that make surgeons mad.

Gum surgery is the last thing you want your dentist to tell you that you need. But that's exactly what Kate's dentist told her.

"I'd really like to avoid it," she said. "The very idea of getting my gums cut makes me queasy."

"You are on friendly turf here," I replied. "Dentistry in general makes me weak in the knees. Maybe that stems from my boyhood, when our dentist didn't believe in Novocain. Gum surgery sounds especially unpleasant."

"They've already scheduled it," Kate said. "They'll do the procedure next month. I'll do it if I have no choice, but I'd sure like to avoid it. Is there any way for me to improve my gums in the meantime?"

"Two things come to mind," I said. "The first is comfrey."

"Is that an herb?"

"Yes," I said, and, spotting a chance to show off, added: "Comfrey has a four-hundred-year history of wound healing. It is favorably mentioned back in Turner's *Herball* of 1568, Gerard's *Herball* of 1597, Parkinson's 1640 *Theatrum Botanicum,* and Tournefort's 1719 *Compleat Herbal.* There have been monographs on comfrey throughout the centuries, and one of the active ingredients, allantoin, is found in salves and lotions today."

"Can I just buy some capsules at the store?" Kate asked.

"Yes and no," I answered. "You can buy comfrey capsules, all right, but they tend to contain dried comfrey leaf. The leaves are best used externally only, and fresh from the plant. Leaves taken internally, as with swallowed capsules, have little benefit, and negative side effects are much more likely. Comfrey, like medicinal herbs in general, is more a medicine than a food. It needs to be used appropriately. The root is what you want, and *the root is not to be taken raw.* Instead, you make a decoction. Basically, a boiled tea."

"And how do you make that?" asked Kate.

"Take a bit of root, maybe a few inches, and wash it under water. Cut the root up, like you would a carrot, into thin slices or little chunks. Put the pieces into a Pyrex or stainless steel saucepan with a cup or two of water. Bring it to a boil, boil for five to ten minutes, and then let it sit and cool. The result is a dark-brown, not particularly unpleasant tea. A cup or two every other day will probably be enough. It can also be used as a mouthwash, and spit out afterward."

"Where do I get comfrey root?" Kate asked.

"Probably at a garden or herb store. I got mine fresh from a farmer who was trying to get rid of it. Comfrey grows like a big weed: very fast. If you mow it down or try to plow it under, it just comes back. Even a little bit of fresh root will grow a new plant. I'm here to tell you, there is nothing to growing your own comfrey. Cheaper that way, too."

"Is that it?"

"Not quite. The second approach you might consider is topical use of vitamin C—direct application of the vitamin to your gums."

"That sounds a bit weird," Kate said.

"It really does," I admitted. "However, vitamin C is so closely involved with wound healing in general and gum integrity in particular that it merits special attention. Vitamin C works as an anti-inflammatory agent. It also is essential for building collagen, the protein 'glue' that literally holds your cells together."

"I'm already taking 1,000 mg of vitamin C a day. Why hasn't that helped?"

"Either it's not enough, or it's not sufficiently concentrated where you need it most."

"But vitamin C is an acid—ascorbic acid, isn't it? I can't go putting that all over my gums and teeth."

"True enough. The trick is to use a nonacidic form of vitamin C called calcium ascorbate. Topical calcium ascorbate will not sting even sore gums, and it is safe to leave on the teeth. You can obtain it as a powder and spread about half a teaspoon on the gum surfaces. It has a bit of a metallic aftertaste, but it's quite bearable. Hold it for about ten minutes, then rinse."

For two weeks, Kate did exactly that, plus drinking the comfrey decoction. However, she did not cancel her gum surgery.

After a pre-op examination, her dentist canceled it.

From time to time I have told my students that, in all honesty, I am not particularly interested in nutrition as a subject. What I am interested in is people getting well, and nutrition is merely the best available means to that end.

Some even believe that. One undergraduate comes promptly to mind. He was twenty-one and suffered from a severe heart arrhythmia. Once every week or two his heart rate would violently soar, his pulse would get erratic, and he'd have to lie in bed for hours before it would return to normal. Sometimes he'd have to lie completely still, quite unable to get up without a recurrence. Occasionally, he'd have to remain motionless for as many as six hours. He was an active fellow, and all this wasted time bothered him as much as the symptoms themselves.

Of course, he'd seen a variety of doctors, including the obligatory specialists. Anxiety or panic attacks had been considered and ruled out. This problem was not in the lad's head. He'd had a lot of tests. The doctors had concluded by offering nothing except either some sort of pacemaker, or a new drug packing the potential of serious side effects. Sitting in my office, he showed me the literature on the proposed drug, and I looked it up.

"This drug might indeed relieve your symptoms, Don," I said. "It can also cause myocardial infarction."

"That's, uh, that's a heart attack, isn't it? I'm way too young to risk a heart attack! And pacemakers are for old guys. There's got to be something else I can do."

"You could try nutrition and see how you do."

His mother had come along to the appointment, and spoke up now. "Nutrition? That couldn't hurt Don. His diet is terrible."

Don gave her one of those classic "Oh, Mom" looks, but that didn't stop her from telling me that he never ate breakfast and chose a lot of junk foods when he did eat. He was also underweight, played a lot of sports, and had a busy work and social schedule. She was plain spoken and pulled no factual punches. She also sounded plenty worried about her boy.

"Let's look at it from the simplest vantage point," I said. "If Don has not been eating well, he should start. If the heart is not well nourished, how could we reasonably expect it to work properly? The heart needs essential fatty acids for fuel. Especially linoleic and linolenic acid."

"I've read about them," said Don's mother. "Aren't they found in fish oil and flaxseed oil?"

"Right. Either source will do."

Don gave a sour look.

"In capsules, Don. Capsules."

He brightened up considerably.

"Vitamin E is next. At effectively large doses, vitamin E helps to strengthen and regulate the heartbeat. It works almost like one of the digitalis family of drugs. You'll need to take a lot, probably over 1,000 IUs daily, perhaps as much as 2,000. You can work up to this level gradually."

"What other vitamins?" asked his mother.

"The B complex and vitamin C would be wise, I think. A variety of cardiac and other muscle problems result from deficiencies in these vitamins. Don may need more of them than the average person. Or maybe his diet has just contained a lot less. I also would follow Dr. Hans Nieper's example and take gram-sized doses of both calcium orotate and magnesium orotate, in about a 2:1 ratio."

And they did try it, cautiously, intelligently, and thoroughly. I had a follow-up session with them not long afterwards. Don was smiling. His mom was smiling. So I smiled, too.

"How's it going?" I asked.

"Great!" said Don. "No sign of any heart problem at all."

Weeks later, we talked again. "I haven't had an attack since I started the vitamins," Don said.

We were all very pleased. I asked Don what he was taking daily, and he read it all off to me: "2,000 mg of vitamin C; 2,000 mg of flaxseed oil; 2,000 mg Calcium orotate in four divided doses; 1,000 mg Magnesium orotate in divided doses; two B-complex supplements; one multivitamin; and 1,600 IU of natural mixed-tocopherols vitamin E."

Not a bad way to eliminate long-standing chronic tachycardia/arrhythmia events so promptly. No pacemaker surgery, no dangerous medicines. It's been a long time now and there has been only one recurrence. That was when Don skipped both breakfast and his supplements. He got back with the program and the symptoms were gone for good.

The simple fact that you are actually reading this says something in itself. Perhaps you have nothing better to do, which I doubt. Or perhaps you have many better things to do, but you can't possibly get on with them until you relieve that itch. Whatever the case, here are my happy-heiney hints:

1. First, we can stop killing sharks (among our newest endangered species). Preparation H and its clones are made from shark liver oil. Use topical vitamin E instead. Medically speaking, "topical" means "applied directly to the surface." This really works, O hemorrhoid sufferers. Make sure the anus is clean and, even more important, dry. After a shower or bath, blot the area with a clean, white tissue and wait ten or fifteen minutes. Then, puncture a vitamin E capsule with a pushpin. (You might even like to keep a pushpin with the bottle, as long as it is out of reach of children and brightly colored so you can spot it, too.) Place the opened end of the vitamin E capsule right up against the anus, and squeeze the capsule. Spread the slightly oily vitamin E around and you will be pleased with the prompt results. Repeat twice daily.

2. Eat more fiber, as found in fruits, vegetables, whole grains, and legumes. This means softer, easier-to-pass stools. Just lovely, this chat we're having here, isn't it?

3. Drink more water. You need water for fiber to work. The bowel is your personal water recycling center, by the way. A human bowel movement usually contains only about 150 ml (that's about half a Dixie cup) of water. The rest, and we're talking quarts, is reclaimed by your body, which is itself two-thirds water. Dry stools are an adaptation for land animals, especially birds and reptiles, to conserve water. Although you are capable of forming a very solid stool, it is better for your butt if you don't.

4. Eat less meat. Meat contains no fiber, and fills you up before you get to the fiber-rich foods.

5. Avoid surgery by doing the four steps above. Some almost personal experience: my dad had several hemorrhoid operations during his lifetime. (He actually watched them perform the surgery, thanks to the wonders of local anesthesia and cleverly placed mirrors. Now there's a lively answer for "What did you do today, Dear?") The simple fact that he had the same operation more than once tells us much about the value of such operations. Dad noted the proctologist's custom-made wallpaper, with its novel,

abstract design. Turns out it was a pattern of assorted anal sphincters. This was in the man's professional office, and I am not making this up: my dad told me. Of course, there is a slim chance that he might have been making it up, and let's hope so.

The rest of this chapter has been pretty much on the level.

There must be *fifteen ways to love your liver.*

1. *Put the six-pack back, Jack.* Half of all the alcohol consumed in America is consumed by only 10 percent of the population. One in three adult Americans is a heavy drinker, with a liquor habit sufficient to be indistinguishable from an alcoholic. Such behavior wrecks livers. Cirrhosis of the liver is a rather rare disease—except among alcoholics, who make it the seventh leading cause of death in the United States! It usually takes half a quart of whiskey a day for ten years to abuse the liver to the point of cirrhosis.

    The fibrous tissue that replaces normal liver in cirrhosis causes decreased liver function. This leads to fluid buildup, jaundice, and perhaps cancer of the liver. Cirrhosis is fairly easy to arrest by stopping alcohol consumption. But cure is difficult and generally considered impossible. Well, as they say in the Marines, the difficult we do immediately; the impossible takes a little longer. Reversing cirrhosis becomes merely very difficult if you employ the Gerson program (referenced below, and in cancer chapters) and very high doses of C and B-complex vitamins. The corticosteroids (Prednisone) are commonly tried for this, but the side effects are undesirable, and in my opinion, the drug is generally ineffective.

    Prevention is the way to go: stop drinking! Sure, as W. C. Fields said, "It's easy to give up drinking; I've done it a thousand times." But consider this: Fields, the highest-paid comic of his time, drank over a quart of hard liquor a day and was dead at age sixty-six.

    That's not so funny.

2. *Avoid the virus, Iris.* The various forms of hepatitis are all diseases that attack the liver, causing symptoms ranging from jaundice, abdominal pain, and diarrhea to nausea, fever, and death. All viral forms of hepatitis respond remarkably well to extremely high doses of vitamin C, the B-complex vitamins, and the Gerson therapy (described below).

3. *Take a lot more C, Lee.* Vincent Zannoni at the University of Michigan Medical School has shown that vitamin C protects the liver. Even doses as low as 500 mg daily help prevent fatty buildup and cirrhosis. 5,000 mg of vitamin C per day appears to actually flush fats from the liver. And vitamin C over 50,000 mg per day results in patients feeling better in just a few days, and actually eliminates jaundice in a matter of days. Frederick Klenner, M.D., found that such huge doses of vitamin C had his patients recovered and back to work in a week.

109

4. *Don't rely on the shot, Dot.* Even if you choose to vaccinate, it is immeasurably reassuring to remember this: Dr. Klenner showed that very large doses of vitamin C (500 to 900 mg per kilogram body weight per day) can cure hepatitis in as little as two to four days.

5. *Take vitamin B, Dee.* Especially vitamin B_{12}, which significantly reduces jaundice, anorexia, serum bilirubin, and recovery time. B_{12} is most effective if administered by injection, which your doctor can easily arrange. If injection is not an option, there is an intranasal gel that improves absorption. Or make your own B_{12} paste (see my chapter "Vitamin B_{12} Supplementation"). This vitamin is nonprescription, utterly nontoxic, and has no contraindications or negative side effects.

6. *Eat veggies and greens, Gene.* The fiber and abundant nutrients in vegetables are a sure way to improve the health of practically any organ you can name, especially the liver. Vegetables are essentially fat-free. And greens are rich in the B vitamin folic acid. (*Folic,* as in *foliage.* Neat, huh?) Folate has been shown to help shorten the recovery time for viral hepatitis.

7. *Eat your food raw, Pa.* Or at least as much of it as you can. Max Gerson, M.D., believed that cancer in general is a disease of the liver, even if it occurs elsewhere in the body. Gerson's nutritional therapy is a raw-foods protocol that is often very effective against cancer, as well as other diseases. Cancer in the liver itself is often due to environmental toxins, such as dry-cleaning fluids. I have personally seen a terminal liver cancer case vastly improved with the Gerson program. Full dietary details are provided in his classic book *A Cancer Therapy: Results of 50 Cases* and in a more recent work, *The Gerson Therapy,* by Charlotte Gerson and Morton Walker.

8. *Get off the drugs, Doug.* Illegal drugs of all sorts (and more than a few prescription drugs as well) are rough on the liver. This includes anabolic steroids. The liver is the main chemical detoxification center for your entire body. Don't push it; quit now before your liver quits on you.

9. *Watch the fat, Matt.* To help relieve indigestion, cut down on those fatty foods. Diseases of the liver can lead to reduced bile secretion. This results in a diminished ability to emulsify fats. ("Emulsify" means breaking down of fat into smaller pieces that can be more easily digested.) Your liver, an enormous four-pound gland, helps you digest fats by normally making up to a quart of bile every day. Most of your body's bile salts are reabsorbed by the intestinal tract after digestion and recycled by the liver. Often, the same bile material will go through two or three recyclings during digestion of a single meal. That is how your body, with less than 4 grams of total bile salts in it, can secrete twice that amount (or more) in a single fatty meal. Gross, huh?

110

10. *Practice safe sex, Tex.* If you are not in a monogamous relationship, you are at increased risk for hepatitis.

11. *Wash your hands, Stan.* Good grief, is that so hard to do? Toilet paper is thinner than a politician's election promise. Do you really think the tissue keeps your hands squeaky clean? To put it another way, do you think it keeps someone else's hands clean enough for you? No? *Then wash your hands with soap and hot water!* I read once that over half of all physicians don't wash their mitts after using the toilet. I hope this is not true. I suspect that it is, however. When heads of state, billionaires, or doctors use the john, they are likely to do what you do. Think about that in your spare time today. And wash.

12. *Prevent that stone, Joan.* In addition to salts for emulsification, bile contains the pigment bilirubin, neutral fat, phospholipids, and high concentrations of cholesterol. About 33 ml of bile are stored in the average gallbladder. But the gallbladder is more than a storage receptacle. It concentrates bile by removing water from it. Sometimes the resulting cholesterol level becomes too high to remain in the bile solution, and cholesterol gallstones precipitate out. In addition to hurting, gallstones obstruct the bile duct, thereby interfering with fat digestion. Low-fat meals help prevent future gallbladder problems by keeping your cholesterol levels low (the body uses fat to manufacture cholesterol). In addition, therapeutic vegetable juice fasting and large doses of vitamin C significantly reduce cholesterol production. This is also an obvious argument for a vegetarian diet, as only animal foods contain cholesterol.

13. *Eat lecithin, Lynn.* Phospholipids in bile help emulsify cholesterol. Lecithin is loaded with phospholipids (also known as phosphatides), to the tune of about 1,700 mg of phosphatidyl choline and 1,000 mg of phosphatidyl inositol per tablespoon. Lecithin therapy is therefore almost certainly worth trying for threatened gallstones. Three to five tablespoons daily is more likely to be effective than a few capsules. Even a large 1,200 mg capsule contains only about $\frac{1}{8}$ tablespoon lecithin because of size limits and added carrier oils. Lecithin is harmless and without side effects. Bulk granules run $8–15 per pound. Lecithin is available over-the-counter at any health-food store.

14. *See your Doc, Rock.* Take the doubt out of it all. Get tested. Be monitored. Listen to your doctor. I said *listen,* not *"obey."* Go and hear what the doctor has to say, and then decide for yourself what you want to do. Negotiation skills and how to shape your doctor into a natural healing practitioner are discussed in other chapters of this book.

15. *Be well-read, Fred.* You can start with the references cited below, and then move on to this book's bibliography.

111

Recommended Reading

Campbell RE and Pruitt FW. The effect of vitamin B-12 and folic acid in the treatment of viral hepatitis. *American Journal of Medical Science* 229 (1955): 8.

Campbell RE and Pruitt FW. Vitamin B-12 in the treatment of viral hepatitis. *American Journal of Medical Science* 224 (1952): 252. [Cited in Werbach, M. *Nutritional Influences on Illness.* New Canaan, CT: Keats Publishing, 1988.]

Cathcart RF. The method of determining proper doses of vitamin C for the treatment of disease by titrating to bowel tolerance. *Journal of Orthomolecular Psychiatry* 10 (1981): 125–32.

Gerson C and Walker M. *The Gerson Therapy.* New York: Kensington, 2001.

Gerson M. *A Cancer Therapy: Results of Fifty Cases and the Cure of Advanced Cancer.* San Diego, CA: The Gerson Institute, 2000.

Jain ASC and Mukerji DP. Observations on the therapeutic value of intravenous B_{12} in infective hepatitis. *Journal of the Indian Medical Association* 35 (1960): 502–05.

Klenner FR. Observations on the dose of administration of ascorbic acid when employed beyond the range of a vitamin in human pathology. *Journal of Applied Nutrition* 23 (Winter 1971): 61–68.

Ray O and Ksir C. *Drugs, Society and Human Behavior,* chapter 9. St. Louis, MO: Mosby, 1990.

Ritter M. "Study Says Vitamin C Could Cut Liver Damage," Associated Press (11 October 1986).

Smith LH, ed. *Clinical Guide to the Use of Vitamin C.* Tacoma, WA: Life Science Press, 1988.

Williams SR. *Nutrition and Diet Therapy,* 7th edition. St. Louis, MO: Mosby, 1993.

You may or may not believe this, but even at the risk of bending the Medical Practice Act, I just had to include it. I got this hiccup cure from my outlaws, er, in-laws, and it is as effective in practice as it is ridiculous in description.

To cure ordinary hiccups, do the following: *Drink out of the far-side rim of a glass.* It may also be described as "drink out of a glass upside down," although you aren't really upside down. Even so, it looks weird enough when you try it.

My experience has been that it takes a full cup of water and about thirty seconds of this type of sipping for the hiccup reflex to cease. It has never failed me. Since I wanted you to gain all possible practical benefit from this book, I couldn't resist mentioning it. (Mag Phos 6X, a Schuessler cell salt in homeopathic potency, is also effective against hiccups.)

A probable explanation for the success of the drinking-out-of-the-other-side-of-the-glass technique is that your bending-over posture and your concentration on performing such an unusual feat serves to restrict the spasmodic inhalation characteristic of hiccups. The act of drinking itself might create new nerve messages to displace the hiccup reflex, calming the glottis and diaphragm. Whatever; it works.

Here's a very common question about a very common problem: "My doctor has recently declared that I have blood pressure that has to be treated and wants to put me on blood pressure pills (the reading was 150/100). Is there a way I can reduce my blood pressure without medication?"

You bet. Switching to a good, near-vegetarian, natural diet would certainly be a good place to start; there is no downside to eating right. More fiber, less sugar and fat, and more fruits, vegetables, and grains are all great for the ticker. So are Dr. Jacobus Rinse's supplement suggestions, which we will come to shortly.

Your BP is significantly higher when you are anxious, and a false reading may result in unnecessary medication. Take your own blood pressure at home, or have a friend do it. You may find that you already have a partial cure for hypertension: avoid doctors' offices! This is more than just rhetorical hyperbole. A daily program of stress reduction repeatedly has been proven to reduce high blood pressure without drugs. (See my chapter "Stress Reduction" for specifics.) Weight loss almost always helps, too. Please look at my chapter on that uncomfortable but important subject.

Back to cardiovascular health in general. Let me tell you about Dr. Jacobus Rinse. When he was only in his early fifties, Jacobus Rinse's doctors told him he had but a few years to live. Cardiovascular disease had ravaged his body. Medicine had little to offer him but hope, and not much of that. So Dr. Rinse, a chemist, decided to look into matters for himself. He hit the books and collected an enormous pile of nutritional research. Some studies suggested that he might be able to delay death with vitamins and other food supplements. He had little to lose, so he tried it. His payoff? Rinse lived for another third of a century.

I drink a modified version of Dr. Rinse's breakfast supplement drink every morning in winter and spring (and juice fresh veggies instead during summer and fall). You can find the recipe for this in my chapter "Breakfast Blast."

My last suggestion, many will note with great joy and considerable relief, has nothing to do with nutrition. Transcendental Meditation is just as effective as prescription drugs for the treatment of high blood pressure. According to a study published in the November 1995 issue of *Hypertension*, TM is twice as effective at lowering blood pressure as is progressive muscle relaxation. Even more important, the results with meditation proved to be just as good as those obtained with pharmaceutical medication. Exactly how good? "Over a three-month interval, systolic and diastolic blood pressure dropped by 10.6 mm Hg." This cannot be written off as a fluke, because a similar study at Harvard yielded the same data: TM for three months reduced systolic blood pressure by 11 mm Hg.

The American Heart Association has said, "People with high blood pressure may want to medicate and meditate." Perhaps they should say it a good bit louder.

Recommended Reading

"In Search of an Optimal Behavioral Treatment for Hypertension: A Review and Focus on Transcendental Meditation" in *Personality, Elevated Blood Pressure, and Essential Hypertension.* Washington, DC: Hemisphere Publishing, 1992.

Rinse J. Atherosclerosis: prevention and cure (parts 1 and 2). *Prevention* (November and December 1975).

Rinse J. Cholesterol and phospholipids in relation to atherosclerosis. *American Laboratory Magazine* (April 1978).

TM combats heart disease. *Vegetarian Times* 221 (February 1996).

Transcendental Meditation, mindfulness, and longevity: an experimental study with the elderly. *Journal of Personality and Social Psychology* 57 (1989): 950–64.

Some physicians would stand by and see their patients die rather than use ascorbic acid.

FREDERICK KLENNER, M.D.

Like a country veterinarian, I drove my red '78 Ford pickup along a vacant road to a client's rural home out near Pavilion, New York. Driving along in the middle of nowhere (and even in New York State there are still such places) to a house call was not my usual routine, but on a sunny spring day like this, it was a taste of the life of James Herriot.

I pulled up the long driveway to the cedar-shingled house where my appointment was scheduled. Going to the side door, I met the father and mother, who showed me into the dining area, where I met a perfectly normal-looking nine-year-old boy. He was blond, fair-skinned, and a bit skinny. His name was Charles.

Charles had no immune system to speak of. His mother told the tale. "He's been in and out of Children's Hospital, again and again. He's home, he gets a sniffle, then he clogs up and can't breathe, then it's pneumonia, then he's back to the hospital. This happens every few weeks, over and over again, and has been going on for years. The doctors said there is nothing they can do except give him antibiotics. They said his immune system isn't working. They do not know why. They are out of ideas, and we are at our wits end over this." She really did look wrung out.

"What can you do?" asked the father. He looked like his nerves were frayed, too. "Nothing has done him any good. All the doctors do is tell us to stick him in a steamy shower when he can't breathe, and we have to keep him there all night sometimes. Then he gets bronchitis. Last time, it went to meningitis."

"Does he take vitamins?" I asked.

"A multivitamin, nearly every day," the mother answered. "Sometimes I give him some vitamin C, but it hasn't helped."

"Maybe his body needs more of it," I said, taking the plunge. "There are fifty years of scientific literature on successful vitamin C megadose therapy. Much of it comes from the two dozen or so published papers of Frederick Robert Klenner, M.D., of Reidsville, North Carolina."

"How much did he use?" the father asked.

"A whole lot; more than you'd ever imagine giving to a nine-year-old."

"We've given Charlie 500 mg sometimes," said his mother.

"Dr. Klenner gave that amount or more per kilogram of body weight per day," I explained. "A kilogram is 2.2 pounds. What do you weigh, Charlie?"

116

"Seventy-five pounds, I think," Charlie said. "Maybe a little less."

"All right, that's about thirty-three kilograms or so. Dr. Klenner would have given you somewhere between 11,000 and 30,000 mg."

"A day?" said his mother.

"Yes."

"That seems like an awful lot of vitamin C," said his father. "How safe is it?"

"Klenner was a very competent doctor, who practiced for some thirty-five years. He wrote that vitamin C is the safest and most effective substance available to the physician. You could start raising Charlie's daily vitamin C intake, and really take it up high if he starts to get sick."

"How high?" asked the father.

"If he gets sick? At least 11,000 mg a day, maybe twice that. Enough so his symptoms stop."

If John Dillinger had told J. Edgar Hoover that he'd never even been in a bank, you could not have gotten a more skeptical look than the one I got then.

"All right, thank you," said the father.

I left without much confidence in this one. It was only days later that I got a call in the morning from Charlie's mother, and she was not happy.

"It's started again," she said. "Charlie is sneezing and coughing and gasping, and we've just put him in the shower. What am I supposed to do again?"

I went over the protocol once more: give Charlie as much vitamin C as he could hold, at least 11,000 mg before the day was over.

"OK," she said. "This had better work."

That's what I was thinking, too. That night I got another call.

"I can't believe it," came the voice of Charlie's mother. "I cannot believe it. He's actually getting better. He's getting better!" She told me that Charlie's symptoms had gone away during the afternoon. He'd had around 12,000 to 14,000 mg of vitamin C that day. No medicines. No more showers. No hospital visit.

"No kidding!" I said. "That's really great."

"Now what?" said the mother.

"As a preventive, continue to keep his vitamin C level high each day, maybe 4,000 mg or so. Dr. Klenner said that children can take their age in grams (thousands of mg) of C each day, as a maintenance dose. My own kids seemed to do fine with around half that. The exact amount will be the amount that keeps Charlie well. Remember that we don't take the amount of C that we think we should take; we take the amount of C that does the job. My corny little jingle is, 'Take enough C to be symptom free, whatever that amount might be.'"

"So when he's sick, give him enough to get him well, and when he's well, give him enough to keep him that way?"

"Right," I replied.

"That seems too simple to be the answer," said his mother.

"The hospital tried everything else, true?" I reminded her.

"Yes."

"And what worked?"

"The vitamin C is the only thing that's worked," she said. "Normally he'd be in the hospital by now. There must be something to this."

There is. And for such a good idea, the spread of this knowledge has been exceptionally slow. Furthermore, for such a useful therapy, medical-political hindrance has been unbelievably high. Nowhere is this more apparent than in the case of Dr. Linus Pauling.

Linus Pauling, Ph.D., is one of history's great chemists, and his textbooks and huge output of scientific papers continue to influence generations of research. Pauling is the only person, ever, to win two unshared Nobel prizes. The first, normally enough, was for pioneering work into the detailed nature of chemical bonds. The second was for peace, after it was eventually appreciated that Pauling's position against atmospheric nuclear weapons testing was the correct one. Neither of these awards prepared the world for what was to follow: Pauling suggested that vitamin C might be effective against the common cold. It would be difficult to imagine that the practical medical applications of ascorbic acid would cause more of a ruckus than Pauling's complete overhaul of our knowledge of chemistry, or the vicious blacklisting Pauling got from the U.S. government when he opposed nuclear testing. But it is true nonetheless.

Pauling reviewed several dozen supposedly open-and-shut papers concluding that vitamin C was apparently unsuccessful at slowing, stopping, or preventing the common cold. He found that the researchers had failed to interpret their own work fairly, or even accurately. In virtually every instance, Pauling found that the effect of vitamin C was, at the very least, statistically significant. Again and again, the authors of the studies had written biased opinions and passed them off as valid summaries of their work.

These authors were simply wrong: science repeatedly demonstrates vitamin C is indeed an effective antiviral. There are other widely known, but completely false, "facts" about vitamin C. Here are two:

Vitamin C Myth #1: "*Your body doesn't absorb extra vitamin C. All you get from taking vitamin supplements is expensive urine.*"

Urine is what is left over after your kidneys purify your blood. If your urine contains extra vitamin C, that vitamin C was in your blood. If the vitamin was in your blood, you absorbed it just fine. Think about that.

You can swallow a marble (but please don't) and find it in the toilet bowl a couple of days later. That is because your food tube, or alimentary canal, is essentially just a twenty-five-foot hose connecting your mouth to your anus. That swallowed marble is "in" your body geographically, but it is not in your body the way your blood is. If you stick your finger through the hole of a donut, you might say your finger is "inside" the donut, but it is not in the donut the way the flour and sugar are. We can turn you upside down and shake you, and you'll probably barf up your most recent meal, maybe even that marble. Your blood won't come out, though. If something is in your blood, it is really in you, fully and utterly absorbed.

If water is coming out of the overflow spillway on a dam, then the reservoir is full and is dumping the excess water. If there is not enough water in the reservoir, nothing comes out. Wasting indicates fullness, just as a cup overflowing is truly a full cup. Urine spillage of vitamin C indicates that you have some to waste, then and there. But such does not indicate bodily saturation; bowel tolerance (loose stool) indicates saturation. Therapeutically, one takes enough C to stay just below that level.

It is the absence of water-soluble vitamins such as vitamin C in urine that indicates vitamin deficiency. If your body excretes vitamins in your urine, that is a sign that you are well nourished and have nutrients to spare. It is easier to put a twenty in the Salvation Army pot at Christmas if you have a few grand to spend shopping. So many Americans are credit-card shoppers and deficit spenders. We are also deficit eaters, trying to obtain a ridiculously low RDA of vitamins from a selection of nutritionally wimpy foods that cannot really meet any of our vitamin or mineral needs abundantly. Vitamin supplements are a solution, not a problem.

Vitamin C Myth #2: *"Vitamin C causes kidney stones."*

I have never seen any scientific evidence to back up that statement. I've had literally hundreds of students and health practitioners looking for years for any controlled study demonstrating a vitamin C–caused kidney stone and so far I have received . . . nearly one submission. In other words, none. The vitamin C kidney stone myth is one of the better-known nonfacts in existence. Every medical doctor has heard of one, yet none of them has ever seen one. Vitamin C does not cause kidney problems; it prevents them (see my chapter "Kidney Disease" for more information).

It's hard to believe that a vitamin can start a scientific civil war, but Pauling speaks from much experience as he discusses this in his exceptionally interesting book *How to Live Longer and Feel Better.* This work, and Lendon Smith's *Clinical Guide to the Use of Vitamin C* (which is about that Dr. Klenner fellow, mentioned earlier) are surely the twentieth century's ultimate treatises on vitamin C "quackery."

I read both Klenner and Pauling. And then I needed them myself, badly. Because I seem to have this little problem with pneumonia.

The first time I had viral pneumonia, I was as sick as a dog. My wife had bronchitis at the same time. We looked so awful that my father took us both to the doctor. The doctor saw my wife first and prescribed Erythromycin, an antibiotic. Then it was my turn. He gave me Erythromycin, too.

"But isn't that useless against a virus?" I asked him.

"Yes. It's for the secondary bacterial infection that often follows the viral infection," he told me. "There's not much we can do about the virus except have you rest in bed."

So I did, knocked silly by codeine cough medicine. For two, perhaps three days, I was in la-la land, not knowing or caring if I ate or not, or if it was day or night. I could barely tell if I was asleep or awake. Nice vacation though it was, neither the codeine nor the erythromycin really cured the pneumonia. The body did, and it took something less than two weeks for me to recover.

The next time I got pneumonia, I did it my way (well, their way) and followed the Klenner/Pauling protocol: take enough vitamin C to get well, no matter how much it may be. This initially makes a lot more sense if you are really, really sick. Pneumonia sets that part up effectively enough.

So there I was, coughing without pause with a fever of nearly 104, playing Scrabble. I literally emptied a bottle of 1,000 mg tablets onto the table, lined them up two by two, and took 2,000 mg of vitamin C every six minutes. In three hours, that amounts to 60,000 mg. And three hours is what it took to lower my fever three degrees and stop my cough completely.

Here's another true confession from my sordid past. I lived off campus as a college senior. Boy, that was fun. Four friends and I closely inhabited one third of a rented house, near the university but well out of reach of the local board of health. We demonstrated our pragmatism, our existentialism, and our sloth on a daily basis. We reduced housekeeping to its most rudimentary form. Plan A: if the dishes in the sink had more than an inch of black mold on them, it was time to clean up. Plan B: forget that, throw them out instead. Plan C: go out for pizza.

Plan C got a lot of use.

We were never sick. Sure, we were young and our immune systems were at their peak. But we were surrounded with germs, as all people are who live outside of a bubble. *This is the whole point:* we live in a world filled with pathogens, but only some of us are sick. There are survivors to every massacre. As a former teacher, I can attest that when the flu comes through school, your absence rate can instantly soar to over one-third of all students. But the other two-thirds, exposed to the same viruses, coughs, and flying phlegm of the school lunchroom, are quite well.

The classic contagious disease would be bubonic plague. The Black Death killed better than one in four Europeans during the fourteenth century. We are talking 30 million people now, plus 45 million more dead in Asia. Pretty awful. Keep in mind, though, that nearly three in four *lived through it.* How? How did the great majority of people *not* die?

It comes down to this: If your immune system is strong (and a strong vitamin-nutritional component therein is indisputable) you will be among the ones who don't get the plague. Or a cold. And if your resistance is down, there is something you can immediately do about it: promptly take vitamin C to saturation, just as those vitamin C quacks recommend.

Vitamin therapy is about curing the real diseases. It is not limited to prevention, and it is certainly not reducible to a few cute platitudes about better food choices. One bold example is a study released in December 1993. At Johns Hopkins, 281 HIV-positive men were studied for six years. Half received vitamin supplements. The other half did not. There were only *one-half* as many full-blown AIDS cases in the vitamin group as in the no-vitamin group. If this were a new *drug* that reduced new AIDS cases by half, it would have been front-page news. But I'll bet that you have not seen one TV, newspaper, journal, or classroom mention of this. And more than 60,000 Americans die each year from pneumonia and the flu. Do you suppose *they'd* have liked to know about vitamin antivirals?

Recommended Reading

Levy T. *Vitamin C, Infectious Diseases, and Toxins: Curing the Incurable.* Philadelphia: XLibris, 2002.

Pauling L. *How to Live Longer and Feel Better.* New York: W. H. Freeman, 1986.

Smith L. *Clinical Guide to the Use of Vitamin C.* Tacoma, WA: Life Sciences Press, 1988.

Kidney diseases kill 60,000 Americans a year and afflict at least 8 million more. Dialysis and transplants are expensive, costing billions of dollars annually. To that, add the emotional and physical costs in pain.

How do your kidneys work? The answer is: constantly! Twenty-four hours a day, your two kidneys filter your blood somewhat like an aquarium filter filters the water in a fish tank. The functional unit of the kidney is the *nephron,* a tissue unit that not only filters, but also recycles and excretes. The nephron cleans the blood, maintains the body's acid-base ion balance, recycles needed substances (water, minerals), and excretes wastes in a concentrated urine. In a manner of speaking, urine is filtered blood, or more exactly, blood is filtered urine. Following are the common diseases with a kidney connection.

Inflammation and Infection

The role of massive doses of vitamin C is profound in the case of kidney infections, providing prevention and treatment at saturation levels. Since vitamin C is filtered and "wasted" through the kidneys, it is a virtually custom-made targeted therapy.

Degeneration

A chronic excess of dietary protein almost certainly taxes the kidneys and leads to gradual degeneration. Reducing protein intake helps prevent the protein-breakdown-induced nitrogenous overload that is responsible. Vegetarianism is the rational solution to this nationwide pattern of protein abuse. Increasing carbohydrates is also recommended to reduce the catabolism of proteins and prevent ketosis. Again, a regular vegetarian diet, which is high in complex carbohydrates, will assure this.

Nephrotic Syndrome (protein in the urine)

This condition results from tissue damage and impaired nephron function. Its association with collagen diseases (such as rheumatoid arthritis) is hardly accidental, for chronic deficiencies of vitamin C (and vitamin C's helpers, the bioflavonoids) cause degeneration of the walls of the kidney's blood vessels, enabling protein to escape into the urine. Capillaries, those tiniest and most numerous of all blood vessels, get leaky in the absence of ample vitamin C. Easily bleeding gums are an example of this. Easily bleeding kidneys need C.

Acute Renal (Kidney) Failure

Early successful management of infectious disease greatly reduces the likelihood of renal failure. Saturation with vitamin C is a very effective, broad-spectrum treatment for infectious diseases. Vitamin C stops the formation of oxalate stones, and actually dissolves phosphate and struvite kidney stones (in the next chapter). If kidney failure is suspected, don't be a martyr: see your doctor early in the game. (Remember, I favor always listening to your doctor, just not necessarily obeying her.) Even conventional nutrition texts mention (correctly) the need for supplemental vitamin C and the B complex for kidney tissue healing. Just up the doses if you want the best results.

In early renal failure, no protein should be given. Vegetable-juice fasting may work well here. If liquids are restricted, put the vegetables through a blender and eat as a salad puree. It tastes better than it sounds.

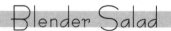

Blender Salad

1 small tomato

1 red or green pepper

$\frac{1}{2}$ small cucumber

juice of $\frac{1}{2}$ lemon or lime

6 leaves romaine lettuce

4 stalks fresh fennel or celery

Cut up tomato, pepper, and cucumber and place in blender. Add lemon juice, and blend until smooth. Add romaine leaves one at a time, to avoid clogging the blender. Add celery or fennel; blend a minute or two longer. The consistency depends upon personal taste; some like it smooth and watery, others thick and crunchy. Eat your blender salad immediately. Crushed raw food does not keep at all.

Chronic Renal Failure

Continued deterioration means loss of vital kidney participation in the activation of vitamin D. The result can be osteodystrophy: calcium deficiency in the bones or poor bone formation during childhood. Supplementation with vitamin D and calcium are therefore required.

Amino acid supplements have shown promise in treating chronic renal failure, when coupled with a greatly curtailed amount of dietary protein of only 20–25 g per day. As an advocate of vegetable juice fasting, I personally think the protein restriction may have done as much as the amino acid supplementation. Why? Because typical hospital "protein-restricted diets" provide 40 g per day of protein!

Consider this: the typical American eats over 100 g of protein per day, and frequently exceeds 120 g, which is *way* too much. So a so-called "restriction" to 40 g per day is simply a correction. Most of the world's peoples would be pleased as punch to be able to eat 40g per day of protein. But we happily chow down three times that, call it normal . . . and then line up for dialysis. The hidden cost of eating meat may ultimately be over $45,000 per year for dialysis. During dialysis, the water-soluble vitamins (B complex and C) are lost from the blood. Supplementation is *essential* and must be both high-potency and frequent.

There are five types of kidney stones:

1. *Calcium phosphate stones* are common and easily dissolve in urine acidi-fied by vitamin C.

2. *Calcium oxalate stones* are also common but they do not dissolve in acid urine.

3. *Magnesium ammonium phosphate (struvite) stones* are much less com-mon, often appearing after an infection. They dissolve in vitamin-C-acidi-fied urine.

4. *Uric acid stones* result from a problem metabolizing purines (the chemical base of adenine, xanthine, theobromine [in chocolate] and uric acid). They may form in a condition such as gout.

5. *Cystine stones* result from a hereditary inability to reabsorb cystine. Most children's stones are this type, and these are rare.

The very common calcium phosphate stone can only exist in a urinary tract that is not acidic. Ascorbic acid (vitamin C's most common form) acidi-fies the urine, thereby dissolving phosphate stones and preventing their for-mation.

Acidic urine will also dissolve magnesium ammonium phosphate stones, which otherwise require surgical removal. These are the same struvite stones associated with urinary tract infections. Both the infection and the stone are easily cured with vitamin C in large doses. Both are preventable with daily consumption of much-greater-than-RDA amounts of ascorbic acid. Think grams, not milligrams! A gorilla gets about 4,000 mg of vitamin C a day in its natural diet. The RDA for humans is only 60 mg. Someone is wrong, and I don't think it's the gorillas.

The common calcium oxalate stone can form in acidic urine whether one takes vitamin C or not. However, if a person gets adequate quantities of B-complex vitamins and magnesium, this type of stone does not form. Any com-mon B-complex supplement twice daily, plus about 400 mg of magnesium, is usually adequate.

Ascorbate (the active ion in vitamin C) does increase the body's produc-tion of oxalate. Yet, in practice, vitamin C does not increase oxalate stone for-mation. Drs. Emanuel Cheraskin, Marshall Ringsdorf, Jr. and Emily Sisley explain in *The Vitamin C Connection* that acidic urine reduces the union of calcium and oxalate, reducing the possibility of stones. "Vitamin C in the urine tends to bind calcium and decrease its free form. This means less chance of calcium's separating out as calcium oxalate." Also, the slight diuretic effect of vitamin C reduces the static conditions necessary for stone formation in general. Fast moving rivers deposit little silt.

Furthermore, you can avoid excessive oxalates by not eating much rhubarb, spinach, or chocolate. If a person is especially prone to forming oxalate stones, they may take their vitamin C in a buffered form. Instead of ascorbic acid, they might use vitamin C as nonacidic "ascorbate." Magnesium, calcium, sodium, and potassium ascorbates are all nonacidic. Other "buffered" vitamin-C preparations are usually made from ascorbic acid mixed with powdered limestone (dolomite). Linus Pauling says you can take a little sodium bicarbonate with ascorbic acid to neutralize it.

Ways for *anyone* to reduce the risk of kidney stones:

1. Maximize fluid intake, especially fruit and vegetable juices. Orange, grape, and carrot juices are high in citrates, which inhibit both a buildup of uric acid and also stop calcium salts from forming.

2. Control urine pH. Acidic urine helps prevent urinary tract infections, dissolves both phosphate and struvite stones, and will not cause oxalate stones.

3. Eat your veggies. Studies have shown that dietary oxalate is generally not a significant factor in stone formation. I would go easy on rhubarb and spinach, however.

4. Skip the soda. Stone-formers are often advised to reduce their calcium intake because most kidney stones are compounds of calcium. Sounds sensible until you think about it. Kidney stones are found in calcium-deficient people. Most Americans are already calcium-deficient (we average only about 500–600 mg of dietary calcium per day, and the RDA is 800–1,200 mg per day). Worse, excess dietary phosphorous causes calcium washout, which we can ill afford. So instead of lowering calcium intake, reduce excess dietary phosphorous by avoiding carbonated soft drinks, especially colas. Soft drinks contain excessive quantities of phosphorous in the form of phosphoric acid. This is the same acid used by dentists to etch tooth enamel before applying sealant.

5. Take a magnesium supplement of at least the RDA of about 400 mg per day. (More may be desirable in order to maintain a 1:2 balance of magnesium to calcium. Some sources even recommend a 1:1 ratio.)

6. Be certain to take a good B-complex vitamin supplement daily that contains pyridoxine (vitamin B_6). B_6-deficiency produces kidney stones in experimental animals and deficiency is very common in humans. B_1 (thiamine) deficiency also is associated with stones.

7. Additionally, a low dietary intake of calcium may itself *cause* oxalate kidney stones.

If there is less calcium in the digestive tract to bind up oxalate on the spot, then there is that much more oxalate to be absorbed and excreted by the kidneys later.

8. For uric acid/purine stones (gout), *stop eating meat!* Nutrition tables and textbooks indicate meats as the major dietary purine source. Naturopathic treatment adds juice fasts and eating lots of sour cherries. Increased vitamin-C consumption also helps by improving the urinary excretion of uric acid. Use buffered ascorbate C.

9. Persons with cystine stones (only 1 percent of all kidney stones) should follow a low-methionine diet and use buffered C.

10. Kidney stones are associated with high sugar intake, so eat less (or no) added sugar.

11. Infections can cause conditions that favor stone formation, such as overly concentrated urine (from fever, sweating, vomiting, or diarrhea). Drink plenty of water. Practice good preventive health care and it will pay you back with interest.

Recommended Reading

Carper J. Orange juice may prevent kidney stones. [syndicated column] (5 January 1994).

Cheraskin E, Ringsdorf M, and Sisley E. *The Vitamin C Connection.* New York: Harper and Row, 1983.

Hagler L and Herman R. Oxalate metabolism II. *American Journal of Clinical Nutrition* 26 (August 1973): 882–89.

Pauling L. Are kidney stones associated with vitamin C intake? *Today's Living* (September 1981).

Pauling L. Crystals in the kidney. Linus Pauling Institute *Newsletter* 1 (Spring 1981).

Pauling L. *How to Live Longer and Feel Better.* New York: W. H. Freeman, 1986.

Smith LH, et al. Medical evaluation of urolithiasis. *Urological Clinics of North America* 1 (June 1974): 241–60.

Thom JA, et al. The influence of refined carbohydrate on urinary calcium excretion. *British Journal of Urology* 50 (December 1978): 459–64.

Williams SR. *Nutrition and Diet Therapy,* 6th edition, chapter 28. St. Louis, MO: Mosby, 1989.

Without showing any slides, photographs or home movies, I'd now like to address a very common question asked of me: "What do you do to keep your family healthy?" People look at my two children, lifelong near-vegetarians, and wonder why they look so good. To a great extent, it is because they are lifelong near-vegetarians! From what I've seen, I'm convinced that eating virtually no meat at all is a tremendous health advantage for children. Our kids were probably the only ones in the neighborhood that had never tasted meat in any form.

When my wife and I started out with our first baby, we didn't know what to do. We'd never been parents before, and we, like you, wanted only the best for our kids. For this reason we decided to raise our children from day one on as natural a diet as possible. We soon realized that this meant breast milk and vitamin supplements for the first six months or so, with the gradual addition of whole-grain cereals, mashed vegetables, fruits, and juices. Now, we didn't know beyond a shadow of a doubt that this would be the best baby diet, but we'd read about it, and we had friends with exceptionally healthy, active, bright-eyed babies who were totally vegetarian. We reasoned that we could always add meat to the children's diet if they really wanted or needed it. So, we decided simply to wait until they asked. They were each about eight years old before they did so.

It is fun to be the parent of little vegetarians. I remember one particular time that I took my three-year-old son shopping at the local supermarket. We passed through the meat department and he pointed to the blood-red packages and loudly asked me, "What's that, Daddy?" I replied, much more quietly, "That is meat." He then declared in a voice that could be heard throughout the store, "We don't eat meat! We're not Italian!" I think he meant to say, "We're vegetarian," but I'm not entirely sure.

Yet another fun aspect of vegetarian children is how happy and healthy the little beezers are. Our children have been much healthier than most children. They missed only a day or two of school a year. We kept a close eye on their health, though, believe me. But aside from the usual colds and such, they were simply healthy. This was largely due to their natural, vitamin-supplemented, virtually meatless diet, in our opinion. What we thought would be best for them has proven in our experience to be best for them. What better evidence is there than success?

The children's good health is owed to the continued grace of God and nature. My wife also gets a lot of credit for having taken the time to feed them right, and also for taking exceptionally good care of herself during both pregnancies. She ate a small amount of meat during the first pregnancy, and less during the second as we both learned more about the benefits of vegetarianism. She also ate a lot of peanut butter, all dairy products, and fish, becoming a near-vegetarian over time. And, of course, she took her vitamins.

Neither of us was raised a vegetarian. As a youngster, I'd attack a hot dog or hamburger just as any other kid would. My wife and I eventually settled on a near-vegetarian diet, meaning we avoided meat and poultry in favor of eggs and some fish, and especially cheese, yogurt, and milk. The point that I'd like to make here is that children do not specifically require meat to get their protein. I'm sure that little children should not be started on meat, and it should not be offered to older kids until they ask for it. And if your home meals are complete without meat, they're not likely to ask.

Perhaps you'd like more details on just how the children ate. Each child got a simple but balanced vegetarian diet consisting of at least two servings each, each day, of corn, beans, and squash. You will remember these as the "three sisters" of the Iroquois. Corn, beans, and squash together make up a complete protein, just like meat, only without the toxins resulting from meat metabolism. However, fear not: my kids didn't live entirely on corn, beans, and squash! They also got dairy products in many forms, especially a wide variety of easy-to-digest cultured cheeses. This was no hardship at all, for they really loved cheese.

For years, their mother baked all of our bread, which was partly but not entirely whole grain, and made with organically grown flours. The children ate peanut butter, walnuts, almonds, and other nuts, ice cream, lots of fruits, all kinds of vegetables, salads, home-baked desserts, casseroles, juices, and pasta (including whole-grain macaroni and spaghetti). They were not finicky eaters, either, for these real foods appeal to children's appetites. Try them on your kids and see for yourself. Start early, preferably in infancy, and you too will have the distinct pleasure of seeing your daughter eat borscht, your son drink lettuce juice, *and your visits to the doctor vanish.*

Each of our children always received a quality multivitamin (liquid, chewable, or tablet, depending on age) twice each day, plus extra vitamin C at each meal. As babies, they had liquid vitamin C, then chewable Cs (which they loved) when they got a bit older. Before they could swallow capsules, every other day they got a few drops of vitamin E (about 50–90 IU) squeezed from a capsule onto their tongue. Believe it or not, they liked the taste of it. It's simple to do, and you can easily control the number of drops you give them. Vitamins A and D, plus the B vitamins, are all in the multivitamin. For kids, choose a multiple preparation containing a natural, chelated form of iron. You can powder a tablet between two spoons and mix it with an infant's pureed fruit. This trick works for vitamin C as well.

We never used fluoridated vitamins, nor did our community have fluoridated water. Our kids have had only a very minimal number of cavities. To this day, my son has only two fillings in his mouth. Always choose vitamins that contain no saccharin, no aspartame, and no other artificial sweeteners. Look for natural flavors, and look to avoid all unnatural additives. We used multiple preparations containing iodine, plus many additional trace minerals.

That's about it, aside from the fact that our children got no brightly colored (meaning artificially colored) "foods" like Jell-O, and no foods containing chemicals including, but not limited to, preservatives. Why feed children paint and poisons?

When our children showed symptoms of a cold or fever, which was seldom, we didn't use medicines, because we have seen that natural methods work better. Knowing that appetites should and do decrease during illness, we switched the kids to a nearly all-fruit diet when illness came on. Think of it as a "kiddie fast." This light, tasty, cleansing diet is very effective for reducing the severity of any illness, naturopaths believe. I would have to agree, and I follow this same plan for myself when I'm not feeling well. The all-fruit diet continues for a few meals or a few days, as long as there's a fever, or sore throat, cough, or runny nose. Remember that these are symptoms of nature's decision to rest and clean the body. A fruit diet is accepted by the children quite easily, for it is just what nature wants them to have at this time. Fruit or especially vegetable juices, their usual vitamin supplements, and lots of extra vitamin C are given throughout the illness.

We monitored sickness in the usual ways with temperature-taking, common sense, and bed rest. *Be sure to consult your doctor for your own situation.* During a fever we didn't give milk or other dairy products, which can be mucus-provoking. High temperature, of course, needs due attention: moderately cool baths (and immoderately high doses of vitamin C) will help lower it. As far as the baths go, Dr. Benjamin Spock in his *Baby and Child Care* standby tells exactly how to do this without aspirin or Tylenol. We ignore the drug parts of the book, and use the rest when needed. *How to Raise a Healthy Child in Spite of Your Doctor,* by Robert Mendelsohn, M.D., is radical but recommended reading for parents with a sick child. For best results, read it in advance.

When your child is sick, you will feel a lot more confident if you keep in personal touch with a knowledgeable, naturopathically oriented physician or teacher, especially at first. Believe me, this is what I did! It's one thing to write a how-to book for other parents; it's another to have that real inner assurance that you're right when it's your own child. The confidence and experience come as you learn by doing. Make it easy on yourself and keep in contact with someone who has been through this before. Someone both supportive and knowledgeable of nature's ways of healing is best. With time you will see your own self-sufficiency, and ability to help healing, grow and grow.

Remember the Four Vs:

1. **V**egetarian diet. 2. **V**egetable juices. 3. **V**itamin supplements.

4. **V**ery liberal quantities of knowledgeable support.

Very effective!

How effective? My son had two visits to a pediatrician in his life, and both were for checkups. My daughter never even met her pediatrician. Yes, we had pediatricians. *The secret is that we never needed them.*

First of all, you probably aren't lactose intolerant, even if you've been told you are. The majority of supposedly lactose intolerant people are not, and can and do eat ice cream and small amounts of milk. A definitive medical test for lactose intolerance is the breath hydrogen assay, which you can have your doctor arrange for you. Only about one in three people initially diagnosed lactose intolerant will turn out to truly be so. I personally speculate that lactose intolerance may be mostly the result of a poor colon bacteria environment, from eating too much of the wrong foods, or even too much of the right foods.

There are several ways to proceed here. First, just avoid milk products completely. Many people simply fare better without any dairy at all. Try for a couple of months and see if you are one of them. Dr. Benjamin Spock (yes, *the* Doctor Spock) recommended against milk, even in growing children. Milks contains lactose, which is digested by the enzyme lactase. Lactase production in humans decreases after age five, and in other mammals not long after birth. A good argument for vegans, perhaps. Be sure you get enough calcium and other bone minerals from moo-less sources such as lots of fresh vegetables. Greens are a great nondairy source of calcium, and whole potatoes are surprisingly good as well. The fruit with the highest calcium content I know of is, believe it or not, the fig! Molasses and almonds are two other ways to bone up without abusing Bossy.

If you are really hooked on the white of the cow (and I confess that this includes me), try limiting yourself to yogurt, kefir, and aged cheeses. These and other cultured milk products are very digestible. Speaking as a former dairyman (I milked over one hundred head twice a day), I will say that fluid milk is perhaps the least desirable dairy product of all, and is also the most likely form to provoke a reaction.

Recommended Reading

Ramig VB. Make your own yogurt. *Mother Earth News Health, Nutrition and Fitness* 11 (1984): 26–28.

Rowell D. What acidophilus does. *Let's Live* (July 1983).

Sandine WE. Roles of bifidobacteria and lactobacilli in human health. *Contemporary Nutrition* 15 (1990).

Savaiano DA and Levitt MD. Nutritional and therapeutic aspects of fermented dairy products. *Contemporary Nutrition* 9 (June 1984).

Sehnert KW. *The Garden Within: Acidophillus-Candida Connection.* Burlingame, CA: Health World, 1989.

Laryngitis

My dad used to say that I learned to talk early and haven't shut up since. Not exactly: I've had laryngitis enough times to look into and find some simple and reliable cures. Here they are:

1. Saturation, or bowel tolerance, of vitamin C will stop laryngitis in a matter of hours. If you take as much C as you can hold, as often as humanly possible, your voice will be back before your friends get to appreciate the silence. People who take megadoses of vitamin C every day preventively are unlikely to ever lose their voice in the first place. When I do weekend seminars, I am speaking for six consecutive hours on two consecutive days. I take about 3,000 mg every hour, and never lose my voice.

2. The homeopathic remedy Ferrum Phos 6X works for loss of voice due either to overstraining or simple inflammation. This remedy works best taken promptly, preferably as soon as you notice the slightest huskiness or hoarseness. A homeopathic remedy is taken until the symptoms begin to improve. Then Mother Nature takes over and your body heals itself.

3. An ounce or two of cider vinegar, straight up, will do wonders for a simple sore throat and laryngitis. When I do this, I get the impression that the vinegar is absorbed into the throat on the way down and never even reaches the stomach. If you immediately, and I mean immediately, follow the vinegar with a "chaser" of an especially sweet fruit juice, you will barely taste the vinegar at all. Be sure to rinse your mouth with water afterward, to remove any lingering acidity. If your stomach is delicate, taking a calcium supplement along with the vinegar will buffer it in the tummy.

4. Avoid dairy products. Dad liked to sing barbershop harmony. Years ago, the men's chorus director (who was also one of my favorite music teachers in elementary school, by the way) told him not to drink milk or eat ice cream before a choral concert. This cannot be just an old wives' tale, because men know of it! Try and see: leave out the dairy if you are going to give us a speech or break into song.

What a beautiful animal the angelfish is. I killed a whole tankful of them with lead, and never knew it.

As a teenager, I was really into tropical fish, successfully breeding Siamese fighting fish at age fourteen. That was a rather strange experience. The babies started to fight at a surprisingly tender age, so of course I had to isolate each one. Until I sold them, I had forty baby-food jars of fighting fish in my bedroom. But they were far from alone; I also kept a large bluegill sunfish (by himself) and an assortment of other species in several more aquariums, utterly filling up my small part of the house. Walking into my room was like a visit to Jacques Cousteau's rumpus room.

I always wanted to breed angelfish. I had a number of really fine angels which I moved to a private tank furnished with some beautiful plants. The plants were held down with some metal "plant weights" that I bought at the local pet shop. Aquatic plants, you see, often get uprooted and float to the surface. So when I saw the package of nice, easily bendable, made-to-order soft metal strips, I bought it.

The weights held the plants down admirably.

All the angelfish died.

It was pretty awful. I woke up one morning bright and early to check on my charges, and half of the angelfish were dead. The rest were swimming erratically, in an unbalanced circling movement. It is sad to see sparkling silver angelfish swimming on their sides, upside down, writhing in their death throes, and not be able to do anything about it.

It was not until I had taken chemistry at college that I realized what had happened. Those plant weights were made of lead. The lead leached into the aquarium water, and the angelfish died of lead poisoning.

Over the years, we have all heard about the hazards of lead. These include lead-paint ingestion by children, lead dust inhalation by miners and metalworkers, lead in solder used in plumbing, and leaded gasoline contaminating cattle. We know that lead poisoning can cause severe mental retardation. Lead has been clearly linked with Alzheimer's disease.

We have been told to avoid lead in the home and to stop lead pollution of our environment. But we have not been told how to remove it from our bodies at home. No drugs are needed; vitamin C megadoses will do the job efficiently. Saturation, or bowel tolerance, doses of vitamin C will snatch the lead right out of a person. That is good news for everybody.

Lead-Avoidance Checklist

Avoiding and removing lead remain the best ways to steer clear of problems with it. The good news is that environmental lead pollution is way, way down, making it one of the great hippie eco-freak contributions to world health. I was there, and saw it happen. The EPA and our much tighter environmental laws are largely 1970s products of 1960s activists.

There is still more to do, though. Here's what is directly in your power:

1. Do not use lead solder for plumbing projects. Make sure your plumber doesn't either.

2. Have lead paint and lead products taken away by your community's Hazardous Waste Disposal Unit. And you do have one; check the phone book's Government Listings, or call the EPA, toll-free, or hit their website, for help.

3. When a lead-painted room, house, or barn is repainted, have the contractor use all precautions, including collection and removal of all paint scrapings.

4. This next suggestion is pretty cool: plant sunflowers. Yes, sunflowers, those giant yellow smiley-faces of the farm, will suck up lead from contaminated soil. Their roots silently clean the dirt as their huge blossoms follow the sun across the sky. I make it a policy to border house, garden, garage, and barn with sunflowers. This is all the more vital if that barn is an old one, and most wood barns are. Each autumn, after the sunflowers dry and die, be sure to throw them out in the trash. Do not burn them or compost them.

The ancient Romans used rot-proof, rustproof, cheap-to-make, easy-to-use lead pipe for their plumbing. In fact, "plumber" comes from the Latin word for lead, *plumbum,* and the chemical symbol for lead remains "Pb" to this day. There is some speculation that the decline of the Roman Empire, complete with its mad emperors, violence, and general dissolution, was the result of chronic lead poisoning.

Fanciful revisionism? Maybe not. Geologic cores in the arctic and elsewhere have shown that the ancient Romans polluted as much as half the world with lead many centuries ago. Smelting metal ores often drives off lead fumes, and they travel with the weather. Autopsies of the corpses of ancient Romans have revealed unusually high quantities of lead in their bodies. They, like my angelfish, never knew what made them sick. Now we know, and we know what to do to get the lead out.

Recommended Reading

Dawson EB, et al. The effect of ascorbic acid supplementation on the blood lead levels of smokers. *J Am Coll Nutr* 2 (18 April 1999): 166–70.

One-quarter of what you eat keeps you alive.
The other three-quarters keeps your doctor alive.
OLD SAYING ATTRIBUTED TO ANCIENT EGYPTIANS.

It is just amazing how tough the human body can be sometimes. Beggars in India were found to have fewer—yes, fewer—dental cavities than well-fed persons in wealthy Western countries. Years ago, one study of 160 beggars found cavities in only two of them. The overall health of the beggars was remarkably similar to that of a comparison group of eighty medical students.

Please do not hurry to catch the next boat to Calcutta, however, just to try to stop Mother Theresa's workers from helping the destitute. The truly poor and the sick need all the help they can get. Still, there is a puzzle here. Is it what the beggars ate, or what they didn't eat, that enabled them to survive in impossible nutrition conditions?

The above study indicated that beggars ate less and were always underfed. And there we may have the answer. The medical students were perhaps overfed, but undernourished, eating more sugar and processed foods. The study also proposed that the beggars had better intestinal flora, or friendly digestive-tract bacteria, to synthesize more of certain B vitamins for them. That would figure, for beggars would receive far fewer courses of antibiotics than "properly" cared for students. At the very least, I think we are left with the suggestion that we should eat less in general, eat less sugar in particular, and eat some more yogurt.

We've tried a few impromptu nutritional experiments in our house. My son had a gerbil that ate fresh seeds, grains, nuts, and garden vegetables. We also fed the gerbil raw bean sprouts. There definitely were times when my son forgot to feed the animal at all. The sleek, shiny, and slim gerbil's name was Mister Chubb, and don't ask why from a boy who invented a dish called "dogstocket." Mister Chubb lived six and one half years. That is very, very old for an animal whose heart beats hundreds of times per minute. Oh, I do wish I'd contacted the *Guiness Book of World Records* on this one, but who would have thought to have certified the birth date of a rodent?

We've also had some rather long-lived cats, and even a catfish that is surely eligible for a pension. The cats get raw egg yolk; what the catfish eats is indescribable. Our dog gets carrot pulp left over from the juicer mixed into her dog food, and has never needed to go to the vet, except to be spayed. My wife raised an amazingly ancient parakeet. It would eat sprouts, too. (Hey, everybody in this family eats sprouts!)

There is, believe it or not, a point to all of this show-and-tell, and here it is: the common thread connecting all these domestic Methuselahs is that we systematically underfed them. I do not mean that they have been starved, but they are seldom allowed to eat their fill. All our pets are a little hungry. In nature, this seems to be the rule by necessity. With pets, and their keepers, it is a healthy rule by design: planned undereating promotes longevity. The best exercise is still to push yourself away from the table. Or the dog dish.

Scientific support for undereating for increased longevity will be found in UCLA Medical School professor Roy Walford's book *Maximum Life Span.* Walford, a medical doctor and distinguished gerontologist, insists that we can live much longer than we'd expect, perhaps to over 120 years of age. This prediction is based on his laboratory experiments that have greatly extended the lifespan of mice, rats, and fish.

And here is the plan: you keep the animals hungry, just like we've been doing at home. Dr. Walford's research found that systematic underfeeding leads to longer lives for animals. And, he submits, it will do the same for people. He calls it "intermittent fasting." You eat every other day, or eat less every day. It's all about "undernutrition without malnutrition." Choosing nutritious foods and taking vitamin supplements are therefore essential. Dr. Walford daily supplements his diet with 1,600 mg of vitamin C and a very substantial 600 IU of vitamin E.

I am pleased that Dr. Walford has openly proclaimed that he takes megadoses of supplemental nutrients. Every medical doctor making such an admission helps patients the world over. Nobel prize winners Linus Pauling and Roger Williams both publicly advocated vitamin supplementation for decades, and both, perhaps not so coincidentally, lived into their mid-nineties.

But the real key to Dr. Walford's plan is what you don't do: eat. This whole topic becomes ever more vital as our years click by. If normal life expectancies are to be believed, my life is already more than half over. Most of us are generally going in the wrong direction: we regularly overeat. Obesity is an epidemic in the United States. And no wonder: in his book, Dr. Walford provides a map of downtown Washington, D.C., showing the locations of no fewer than sixty-four food lobbyists' offices—all within a few blocks of the White House.

The idea that the long-sought Fountain of Youth may consist simply of undereating is pretty wild. But then, think of the money you'd save. Think of the years you'd gain.

Those beggars in the India study would almost surely have been healthier with a better balanced diet and vitamin supplements. I think we all would be. But with many vitamins, the B-complex in particular, deficiencies can actually rise with unhealthy food intake. If you avoid unnecessary calories, your vitamin need can decline. This also means that if you overeat, your vitamin need is going to be higher. Unfortunately, just eating more of the standard American diet of empty calories from foodless foods does not provide healthy quantities of vitamins. Eating more of the wrong thing is no solution.

The Best Health and Longevity Bargains Ever

1. The don't-stuff-yourself vegetarian diet, or as close as you can get to it.

2. The high-potency, natural multivitamin-multimineral supplement, twice daily.

3. The use of extra vitamin C and extra vitamin E daily.

4. Eating lots of raw foods (like salads and sprouts) and fresh raw vegetable juices.

Medical and nutritional research supports this plan. So do the experiences of millions of vegetarian or near-vegetarian Americans who take vitamin supplements each day. So does our family's pet menagerie. And, I am happy to say, our kids prove it, too. Whenever I give a nutrition lecture, people listen to me but want to see my kids. So sometimes I tote them along as exhibits. I suppose I could take some pets instead, but the kids answer questions better.

Recommended Reading

Pathak CL. Nutritional adaptation to low dietary intakes of calories, proteins, vitamins and minerals in the tropics. *American Journal of Clinical Nutrition* 6 (March–April 1958): 151–58.

Walford RL. *Maximum Life Span.* New York: W.W. Norton, 1983.

Ménière's Syndrome and Tinnitus

It shook me deeply to see my father have to crawl to the bathroom to vomit. Dad was only in his mid-fifties and was already using a cane to stand up, when he could stand at all. He had a really bad case of Ménière's syndrome, a miserable collection of symptoms including recurrent ringing in the ears, dizziness, and nausea. Perhaps it was a defining moment for me. Seeing your father reduced to helplessness is enough to make anyone want to know more about getting well. When you look this one up, the treatments you come across, whether pharmaceutical or surgical, are primarily aimed at the symptoms, because the cause of the illness is pretty much unknown.

Enter natural healing. By trial and error, I have found some drugless, scalpel-less options for Ménière's. While the solutions may shed some light on the cause, I, like you, am interested in results.

Chiropractic or osteopathic adjustment of the upper cervical (neck) vertebrae is worth trying. Some twenty years ago, I met a young man so dizzy that he could not read or even watch TV without having to lie down. Ménière's, aptly described in the *Merck Manual* as "prostrating," certainly is capable of flooring a person. Such was the case with Lowell, a college dropout. He had a gentle but persistent series of chiropractic manipulations that restored his life. He was able to read again, to return to school, and to live again. How so? The practitioner discovered that his two top neck vertebrae, the atlas and the axis, were practically at right angles to each other, and to the skull as well. This seemingly impossible state of affairs turned out to be due to a summer job Lowell had a few years before: he was a sparring partner for boxers in training. He had almost literally had his block knocked off.

Pa refused to go to a chiropractor until his Ménière's was so bad he could not take it any more. He'd been on various ineffective medications from various ineffective physicians, none of whom gave chiropractic the time of day. But I managed to get him to a D.C. for a visit or two. Pa said it did not help one bit.

He then began taking vitamins, notably the B complex in fairly high doses. Pa had no praise for that, either. But over a period of months, his specialist-diagnosed Ménière's went away.

I had persistent suspicions that the natural approach helped him.

Since then, I have come across references showing that **niacin** has been used for Ménière's syndrome since the 1940s. In long-term therapy, improvement has been obtained with only 150–250 mg daily. This may explain why Pa's improvement was so gradual, yet in the end, profound.

I think that Ménière's syndrome, and perhaps a number of other difficult-to-tag neurological problems, could be a manifestation of untreated, long-term **B₁₂ deficiency**. I discuss this, and what to do about it, in my chapter "Vitamin B_{12} Supplementation."

The late Lendon Smith's newsletter *The Facts* mentions that **aspartame** ("Nutrasweet") may "trigger or mimic" a Ménière's attack. Dr. Smith specifically lists nausea, vertigo, hearing loss, and tinnitus as symptoms that say, "Stop using aspartame."

A **low-fat, low-sodium, no alcohol, and especially *no sugar* diet** may help a wide variety of illnesses. Ménière's seems to be closely connected with chronic low blood sugar, sometimes diagnosed as hypoglycemia or type 2 diabetes. Caffeine may aggravate the condition, as might manganese deficiency.

Zinc supplementation and moderate additional amounts of B_6 (pyridoxine) are also worth a several-month therapeutic trial.

For uncomplicated simple ringing in the ears, dizziness, or nausea, a 6X potency of **Kali Phos** (a homeopathic remedy) may be surprisingly helpful. I have personally used this remedy for thirty years, as I have a motion-sickness problem that my flight instructor insists he's never seen topped. If it were not for Kali Phos, not only would I not have passed my flight test, I think I would have thrown up right in the FAA examiner's lap directly over the Batavia, NY airport.

My Dad, fully recovered from Ménière's, walked four miles a day for the rest of his life. His dizziness and nausea were gone for good. His sense of humor was not, however. If you ever asked my father how his hearing was, he'd invariably shout back at you, "WHAT?" But he did it smiling, and standing up straight.

Recommended Reading

Balch J and Balch P. *Prescription for Nutritional Healing.* Garden City Park, New York: Avery, 1990, 239–40.

Bicknell F and Prescott F. *The Vitamins in Medicine,* 3rd ed. Milwaukee, WI: Lee Foundation, 1953, 379.

Werbach M. *Textbook of Nutritional Medicine.* Tarzana, CA: Third Line Press, 1999, 475–82.

Menopause has been medicalized into a disease. It is not. Just as menarche (the start of menstruation) is a natural process, so is its cessation also a natural process. The symptoms we associate with menopause still need to be addressed, of course, but perhaps from a slightly different angle.

It is interesting that the medical profession, which is set against treating vitamin deficiency with vitamin supplements, has no difficulty treating hormonal deficiency with hormonal supplements, even though estrogen supplementation carries significant risks.

Women taking estrogen-progestin therapy have increased incidence of heart attack, stroke, dementia, ovarian cancer, and breast cancer. Consequently, I think estrogen/progesterone replacement, supplements, or creams are not a good idea. To me, even the natural-source products raise a caution flag. The body's hormonal system is a beautifully (if delicately) balanced one, and not to be messed with. If you gave me a new Porsche, and I went under the hood with a wrench, I could only do harm. The same with your endocrine system.

On the other hand, frequent oil changes, good gas, safe driving, and lots of preventive maintenance can really prolong the life and beauty of a car—or a woman. For the human body, such a systemic approach is best done through nutrition. It is a popular myth that a woman's endocrine system self-destructs the moment she stops ovulating. It doesn't. It is still there, and it still works. Feed it right and many a "menopausal symptom" bites the dust.

Here is an asssortment of potentially helpful suggestions collected by a guy who has, at least so far, only experienced menopause secondhand.

Hot flashes and night sweats: vitamin E, 800 IU or more per day, and vitamin C to saturation as described in my chapter "Vitamin C Megadose Therapy," plus supplemental linolenic acid.

Constipation: vegetable juicing is the world's best cure for this.

Dizziness and headaches: chiropractic, and the homeopathic remedy Kali Phos 6X. (See my chapter on Meniere's syndrome.) Strictly avoid caffeine, aspartame (Nutrasweet), sugar, and alcohol.

Fatigue: vitamin C, and plenty of it. (See my chapter "Vitamin C Megadose Therapy.")

Heart palpitations: magnesium (400–600 mg) and calcium (1,000 mg), especially as orotate or aspartate. The citrate form is okay. Calcium supplementation with 1,000 IU/day of vitamin D will also help prevent osteoporosis.

Irritability, anxiety, or insomnia: high-tryptophan foods such as cashews, plus lecithin (several tablespoons daily) and niacin. (See my chapters "Saul's Super Remedy" and "Sleep Disorders.")

Vaginal itching and dryness: vitamin E topically may help. The natural form is best. Use water-based lubricants for intercourse.

Hypoglycemia: B-complex supplements, with each meal and between each meal. Be sure to increase your dietary fiber. Eat no sugar, but lots of raw veggies, cooked brown rice and beans, and whole grains. Chromium (200–400 mcg daily) is also a wise addition.

Stress Reduction: exercise, meditation, yoga, and similar techniques are very valuable. (See my chapters "Stress Reduction" and "Avoiding Exercise.")

Recommended Reading

Balch J and Balch P. *Prescription for Nutritional Healing.* Garden City Park, New York: Avery, 1990, 241–42.

"U.S. Studies: More Bad News for Hormone Replacement Therapy." Reuters Health, May 27, 2003.

Americans generally do what their doctor tells them without many questions. I suggest they question their doctor extensively, and not necessarily do what he says. Then hit the books for a really different second opinion.

And if someone has multiple sclerosis? The answer, and it is a remarkably good answer, is to follow the MS protocol of Frederick Klenner, M.D., as described in *Clinical Guide to the Use of Vitamin C,* edited by Lendon Smith, M.D. Far from just considering vitamin C, this book urges and lists a comprehensive therapeutic program using a large variety of nutrients in significant quantity. Here are Dr. Klenner's most important nutrient recommendations for MS (which also apply to myasthenia gravis, a disease involving the neuromuscular junction), all of which should be divided up throughout the day:

- Vitamin B_1 (thiamine): 1,500–4,000 mg per day, orally and by injection

- Vitamin B_2 (riboflavin): 250–1,000 mg per day

- Vitamin B_3 (niacin): 500 mg up to many thousands of milligrams daily, enough to cause repeated episodes of warm-feeling vasodilation ("flushing")

- Vitamin B_6 (pyridoxine): 300–800 mg per day

- Vitamin B_{12} (cobalamin): 1,000 mcg three times a week by injection

- Vitamin C (ascorbic acid): 10,000–20,000 mg per day

- Vitamin E (d-alpha-tocopherol): 800–1,600 IU per day

- Choline: 1,000–2,000 mg per day

- Magnesium: 300–1,200 mg per day

- Zinc: 60 mg per day, taken with meals

- Calcium, lecithin, folic acid, linoleic and linolenic acids, and a daily multi-vitamin-multimineral tablet supplement are also recommended

Why such a large variety of nutrients? Because there is no such thing as monotherapy with nutrition. "One drug, one disease" is a failed legend of the drug doctor. People often ask me, "What is this vitamin good for?" My answer is, "Everything." They give me the look, but it's true nevertheless. All vitamins are important. Which wheel on your car can you do without? Which wing on an airplane can you afford to leave behind?

Why large quantities of nutrients? Because that's what does the job. You don't take the amount that you think should work; you take the amount that gets results. The first rule of building a brick wall is that you have got to have enough bricks. A sick body has exaggeratedly high needs for many vitamins. You can either meet that need, or whine about why you didn't.

But why try to cure with nutrition? Well, why not? Must a cure be medical for it to be any good? There is no medical cure for MS; if there were, you would have heard about it. I say, if one doctor's black bag is empty it does not necessarily follow that all other doctors' black bags are. Go where you can get the outcome you need. The first rule of fishing is to put your hook in the water, for that is where the fish are.

Let's consider just one lone nutrient, thiamine, and one oddball disease, beriberi. Beriberi has been a problem for centuries in impoverished countries. It is a disease of the peripheral nervous system. Beriberi, the very description of nutritional exhaustion, literally means "I can't, I can't." It results in pain and paralysis, swelling and anemia, decreased liver function and wasting away. Note, please, the wide variety of symptoms.

No drug on earth, then or now, can cure it. For centuries, the question has been: what exactly causes it? In 1897, Dr. Christian Eijkman first cured beriberi. He had previously observed that many prisoners had the disease. They were fed a diet dominated by polished (white) rice, the stuff Americans eat to this day. Eijkman fed the prison diet to pigeons and watched the same beriberi symptoms emerge. He then fed the sick pigeons unmilled (brown) rice. The birds were cured. He tried whole brown rice on the prisoners, and they were cured. Completely. No drug had done that; it took brown rice, and something special in that unprocessed rice. Eijkman later received the Nobel Prize for this work.

143

In 1911, Casmir Funk, a Polish chemist living in London, would discover that special something in the outer, usually wasted rice hulls. Because it was a nitrogen compound, he labeled it an amine. Because it was vital to health, it was a vital amine, or vitamine, or vitamin. The name stuck and became generic, like Kleenex.

Between 1909 and 1916, the Philippines-based American R. R. Williams began curing beriberi in young children with outstanding success. The rice polishings he used were thereafter called vitamin B (for beriberi?) and thought to provide a single essential chemical. Today known to be a team of vitamins, the B complex (as well as vitamin C) are all water-soluble, indispensable, and generally not stored by the body.

Thiamine helps form a coenzyme needed in glucose oxidation to either get energy from glucose or to produce fat (which is called lipogenesis). Without thiamine, these do not occur. At all. Hence, the fatigue and wasting away of beriberi. The mineral magnesium is another essential factor in this process.

Thiamine is not stored in tissues. You need it every moment of every day, and it plays a crucial role in carbohydrate metabolism, pregnancy, lactation, and muscular activity. Less well known is that more thiamine is needed by the body's tissues during fevers.

A long-standing inadequate thiamine supply may cause severe neurological effects, most significantly nerve irritation, diminished reflex response, prickly or deadening sensations, pain, damage to or degeneration of myelin sheaths (the fatty nerve cell insulation material), and ultimately paralysis. Dr. Klenner, aware that this could well describe multiple sclerosis, went to work trying megadoses of thiamine. On the principle that it takes a lot of water to put out a well-established fire, Klenner ignored the RDA of 1–2 mg per day and gave MS sufferers thousands of milligrams of thiamine per day. He administered other vitamin megadoses as well. Patients improved.

That book again? *Clinical Guide to the Use of Vitamin C.* It is out of print, but you might be able to obtain a used copy over the Internet. If you cannot find the book, just read Klenner's studies individually. You can do a search at any library, and then get a copy of each of his papers through interlibrary loan. And without a prescription, too.

Recommended Reading

Smith LH. *Clinical Guide to the Use of Vitamin C.* Portland, OR: Life Sciences Press, 1988, 42–53.

Medical scientists have spent the last few hundred years carefully describing diseases that are in reality the end results of chronic malnutrition. Researchers have expended colossal amounts of time and money searching for drug cures for nutritional disorders. And they have dismissed out of hand even the possibility that pharmaceutical therapy for malnutrition might be the dead end it has so frequently been shown to be.

Parkinson's disease is a case in point. L-dopa (levodopa) is a commonly prescribed treatment for Parkinson's. The human body can make this substance without drug intervention. Vitamin C in very high doses greatly stimulates L-dopa production, as well as enables your body to naturally and safely produce its end product, the neurotransmitter norepinephrine. A depletion of norepinephrine may result in poor memory, loss of alertness, and clinical depression. The chain of chemical events in the body resulting in this substance is:

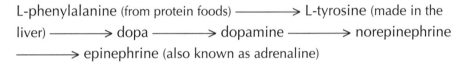

L-phenylalanine (from protein foods) ⟶ L-tyrosine (made in the liver) ⟶ dopa ⟶ dopamine ⟶ norepinephrine ⟶ epinephrine (also known as adrenaline)

This reaction chain looks complex but actually is readily accomplished, particularly if the body has plenty of vitamin C, which facilitates the process. Since one's dietary supply of the first ingredient, L-phenylalanine, is usually adequately provided by protein foods, more likely a shortage of vitamin C is what limits production of norepinephrine. Physicians giving large doses of vitamin C have had striking success in reversing depression. It is a remarkably safe and inexpensive approach worth trying for Parkinson's.

Another important neurotransmitter, acetylcholine, can be made by your body from dietary choline. Choline is obtainable in quantity, and at low cost, from supplemental lecithin. Acetylcholine is the end neurotransmitter of your parasympathetic nerve system, which is responsible for, among other things, good digestion, deeper breathing, and slower heart rate. You may perceive its effect as "relaxation."

Lecithin is found in egg yolks and most soy products. Three tablespoons daily of soya lecithin granules provide about 5,000 mg of phosphatidyl choline. Long-term use of this amount is favorably mentioned in *The Lancet* (February 9, 1980). Lecithin supplementation has no known harmful effects whatsoever. In fact, your brain by dry weight is almost one-third lecithin! How far can we go with this idea of simply feeding the brain what it is made of? In *Geriatrics* (July 1979) lecithin is considered as a therapy to combat memory loss. Studies at MIT showed increases in both choline and acetylcholine in the brains of animals after just one lecithin meal.

So, rather than give a synthetic drug to block or mimic the body's chemical nerve messengers (neurotransmitters), it is possible nutritionally to encourage the body to make its own natural ones. If these seem impossibly simple solutions for so dreaded a disease, you are left with a simple cost-benefit question: Since no one dies from vitamin C or lecithin, why not try them? Exactly what do you have to lose? Or, perhaps, regain?

People with Parkinson's will also do well to embrace a low-protein diet. Mostly-raw-food vegetarianism is the simplest way to accomplish this. Do not be dissuaded by this low-tech but important option.

Recommended Reading

Werbach, M. *Nutritional Influences on Illness.* New Canaan, CT: Keats Publishing, 1988.

Werbach, M. *Textbook of Nutritional Medicine.* Tarzana, CA: Third Line Press, 1999.

She was a really cute, really curly-haired ten-year-old girl, and she was really dying. She knew it, her Mom knew it, and her doctors told them so. Her name was Patty. Patty's body was destroying her platelets faster than she could make new ones. Platelets are specialized blood cells that are responsible for clotting blood. Hospitals full of specialists had studied this girl and her rare problem. They concluded by telling her mother that they had tried everything, and there was nothing else to do.

So, Patty's mom brought her to see me. The quack.

Patty knew more about her illness than I did. I still don't know the proper medical name for it, and it doesn't much matter. She was a cheerful, calm, bright, personable little thing, and this was in tremendous contrast to her gaunt, wired mother. The mother had passed the point of mere panic long ago; she was desperate.

"We've tried everything," the mother said. "She's had all the tests. She's seen all the specialists. Nothing helps. Her platelet count is less than one-tenth of normal, and keeps dropping every week. What can be done? Can you help her?"

I didn't know. So I sat down and talked to Patty. "Do you understand your illness, Patty?" I asked. She nodded. Then she proceeded to tell me all about it. I listened, and came up with an idea. "There is at least one thing the doctors have not tried," I said. "Vitamin C and vitamin K are necessary for platelet production. It is a long shot, but maybe Patty's body needs more of these vitamins—far more—than other people do. You can megadose her on vitamin C easily enough, as it's nonprescription, cheap, and safe. You can get vitamin K from alfalfa sprouts, like the ones you see at salad bars and supermarkets."

They looked back at me. The mom eventually asked, "How much does she need to take?"

"I'm not sure, but probably a lot. It's pretty hard to hurt yourself with sprouts, and guinea pigs have been given the human dose equivalent of half a million mg of vitamin C a day without harm. You could try 10,000 mg a day. If Patty takes too much, she'll get loose bowels. If she were my daughter, I'd have her eat all the sprouts she can hold. If she eats too much alfalfa, her blood will clot too easily."

"That would be a nice problem to have!" Patty said, and her mom actually smiled.

I heard from the mother about two weeks later, and I was nervous when she started speaking. "Patty has been eating one to two jars full of alfalfa sprouts a day. She's been real good about it. And she's been taking the 10,000 mg of C every day as well."

"And?" I asked.

"The doctors have seen her several times, and her platelet count is now 85 percent normal. She is going to live! I'm so thrilled!" And off she went for a while, talking of how wonderful this all was. Inevitably, she came to the question that I've heard a thousand times. "So why didn't the doctors try this?"

It's a good question, isn't it? You can usually find only what you are looking for. There are famous exceptions, and Columbus comes immediately to mind. He was looking for India and bumped into an entirely different continent. At least explorers are usually listened to when they return with their first-hand accounts of discovery. You should see what happens to unorthodox health practitioners, and scientists, and medical doctors too, when they "discover" that vitamins cure real diseases. One of the first things that happens, as they gracefully lose their reputations, is that they are forever labeled quacks.

Patty does not care about any of that. She lived, and that's enough.

Do you remember when there wasn't even a name for what we now know as PMS? It wasn't that many years ago that doctors considered it to be all in a woman's head. Long before that, "hysterical" women were considered to have it all emanating from their uterus. The solution? Surgery to remove the uterus (and with it the hysteria), hence the term *hysterectomy*. Half a million hysterectomies are still performed annually, most of them medically unnecessary.

Even twenty years ago, I do not recall much serious discussion about PMS. A lot of angry ladies changed that. Now TV ads discuss PMDD (premenstrual dysphoric disorder). What's a dysphoric? A person exhibiting dysphoria, of course. Now for the real answer: a person with anxiety, depression, and restlessness.

So now I've got dysphoria to read. (That was subtle, but did you get it? If you didn't, I'll get datphoria next time.) But seriously, folks, many cases of PMS/PMDD can be relieved through vitamin B_6 and magnesium supplementation. Let's explore each.

Vitamin B_6

PMS/PMDD symptoms are greatly relieved by vitamin B_6 supplementation. Depressed persons are commonly deficient in this vitamin, which is necessary for your body to make the neurotransmitter serotonin. Serotonin is that wonderful feel-good substance that SSRI drugs such as Prozac try to maximize in your brain. If B_6 can do the same thing, at a fraction of the price, it is no surprise that there have been attempts to discredit its use.

B_6 dosage to the tune of 500 mg per day is generally very safe. Probably tens of millions of women suffer PMS symptoms; very few cases of B_6 overdose have been reported. High daily dosage (usually over 2,000 mg) has occasionally caused temporary neurological symptoms in some people. But as a rule this only happens if it is given alone, or way out of proportion to the other essential B vitamins. Taking all the B vitamins together (as B complex) is the safest and most effective therapeutic approach. When a balance is maintained, B-vitamin toxicity is virtually nonexistent. Is there a safe harbor? I think so. Use the entire B complex, taken every two to three hours. Consider adding perhaps 50–100 mg of pure B_6 to each dose if dysphoric symptoms are really awful.

You can get some (probably less than 5 mg) B_6 from food, if you really like to eat whole grains, seeds, and organ meats. A goodly slice of beef liver contains a whopping 1.22 mg of B_6. Other dead animal parts contain less (turkey and chicken breasts are pretty good, but chicken liver is only 0.6 mg per serv-

149

ing), while most other foods contain very little. Avocados (0.5 mg each) and bananas (0.7 mg each) lead the pyridoxine league for fruits. Potatoes (0.7 mg each) and nuts (especially filberts, peanuts, and walnuts) are relatively good veggie sources.

The RDA for B_6 for women is 1.6 mg daily, which is ridiculously inadequate. A strong case can be made for increasing this to at least 25 to 65 mg per day for people without PMS symptoms. But don't hold your breath for a raising of standards anytime soon. It seems to be hard enough to get people in the United States just to meet the RDA. Consider that about three-quarters of children ages 2–12 do not get the RDA of B_6. That's pretty terrible, but it is worse for adults 19 and over: 99 percent get less than the RDA of B_6. That goes a long way to explaining the prevalency of the PMS problem.

Magnesium

"Increasing dietary magnesium often decreases menstrual cramping associated with PMS. While calcium is also important for normal muscle function, magnesium can specifically help them to relax. Lots of women take extra calcium, which may help relieve cramping, and certainly has bone benefits. However, supplemental calcium alone effectively depletes the body of magnesium and ensures cramping will occur in the following month if magnesium is not replenished.

"If you do not suffer from kidney disease, consider taking an oral daily magnesium supplement. For generally healthy people the only significant side effect from taking too much magnesium is diarrhea. Your body continuously discards excess magnesium through urine and feces.

"The RDA for magnesium is 420 mg per day for men and 320 mg for women. This standard may be inadequate, and, what's worse, the majority of people do not get even that much. Magnesium is necessary for the normal functioning of more than three hundred enzymes in your body. If you do not have enough available magnesium (magnesium deficiency), it slowly degrades your general health in a variety of ways. Magnesium deficiency is directly linked to heart disease. Moreover, because of the many ways your body employs magnesium, it plays a role in preventing diabetes, cancer, stroke, osteoporosis, arthritis, asthma, kidney stones, migraine, leg and menstrual cramps, eclampsia, PMS, chronic fatigue syndrome, tetany, and a variety of other problems.

"Magnesium supplements are inexpensive and readily available without prescription. Women might try starting with 200 mg per day, divided up into two or three separate doses. After two weeks, you can increase your daily dose by a convenient increment, say 100 mg per day (tablets are easily snapped in half). If frequent bowel movements or gas become a problem, reduce the amount." (From "The Role of Magnesium in the Prevention of Coronary Disease and Other Disorders," by Tom Miller. http://www.mgwater.com/tmiller.shtml. Reprinted with permission.)

Recommended Reading

Seelig M. *Magnesium Deficiency in the Pathogenesis of Disease.* New York: Plenum, 1980.

The best possible preparation for pregnancy is a lifetime of good nutrition. This is especially true during the years immediately preceding conception. In a manner of speaking, a baby is nearly a year old at birth. Many women only begin to eat right and take necessary vitamin supplements once they confirm they are pregnant. This is weeks or even months too late. The first few weeks of pregnancy are especially crucial to the embryo.

Let's steel ourselves to take a quick look under the bed at what every parent-to-be is most terrified of: the uncomfortable subject of birth defects. Here is a grim fact from the National Institute for Drug Abuse: Fully 11 percent of all babies born in the United States are born to drug-abusing mothers. Here's another: Mothers who smoke tobacco are hurting their unborn child. The carcinogens and other harmful chemicals that a pregnant woman takes in when she smokes cigarettes are transmitted to the unborn baby. Many chemicals in tobacco products, such as benzene and formaldehyde, are known teratogens (causes of birth defects).

Maternal alcohol use also hurts the developing child. Two out of three adults use alcohol, and one in ten adults is a heavy drinker. The Surgeon General has stated that *there is no safe minimum level of alcohol consumption during pregnancy.* Fetal Alcohol Syndrome is the most severe expression of what alcohol can do to a baby. There must be millions of infants with less obvious but still handicapping alcohol-related congenital damage.

In addition, environmental pollutants and on-the-job exposure to chemicals are causes of birth defects. And we have not even considered pharmaceutical side effects (remember thalidamide?). Then there is malnutrition, or undernutrition, which may be the greatest factor of all. I would be willing to say that the majority of pregnant women strictly avoid harmful behaviors. But there are others who persist in doing multiple dangerous behaviors well into, or throughout, pregnancy. This constitutes child abuse, and it must stop immediately, before it is too late.

Along with chemical abuse, poverty and extremes in maternal age traditionally make up the common problem pregnancy areas. Bottle feeding, unnecessary overmedication, and marginal nutritional deficiency diseases make up three additional problem areas. For a really bone-chilling summary of the consequences of vitamin deficiency during pregnancy, read the papers by Howard Hillemann referenced below.

Nutrition needs rise during pregnancy, of course. Even the RDAs are higher. This may be obvious to you, but many women eat poor diets in general. They then tend to eat more of the same lousy foods in an attempt to "eat for two" and "to get all the nutrition they need from a balanced diet." This is a genuine tragedy, for which the medical and nutrition professions cannot easily be excused. At the very least, pregnancy increases the need for protein, calcium, iron, and all of the vitamins. The same for lactation. And don't forget Dad: conception is more likely if Dad takes supplemental vitamin C, zinc, lecithin, and a little Korean ginseng extract (*Panax ginseng*) each day. See my chapter on fertility for more information.

Ten Ways to Avoid Most Birth and Baby Problems

1. A pair of really hip obstetrical nurses taught me that pain is a function of tension, particularly during childbirth. Try meditation to reduce stress and tension. (See my chapter "Stress Reduction.")

2. Avoid drugs of all kinds: alcohol, cigarettes, illegal drugs, and all but the most essential medications.

3. *Nurse your baby from day one!* Did you know that breast milk actually changes composition to meet the needs of the developing baby? For example, preemies actually get a higher-protein, higher-fat milk than full-term infants. There is apparently a very sensitive and complex relationship between the physiology of the mother and baby after birth, as well as before. Colostrum immunity is an important part of this. Breast milk changes again during later nursing and during weaning, supplying still more protein and, yes, some iron. Do not supplement with formula: the breast, or the udder for that matter, makes more milk when demanded of it. Ladies, if you use formula "also," you will start to make even less milk. A spiral will develop, resulting in no more breast milk. I am forever grateful to my sister-in-law for telling my wife to just "put the kid on the breast and suffer with it for a day or two. There will be more milk, don't worry." She was right. I remember the baby virtually drowning in milk after that. Make a point to read *The Womanly Art of Breastfeeding*, by the La Leche League International. This is a good, good book.

4. Take vitamin A as carotene. Is it safe, you ask? Let's talk polar bears, shall we? Since three-quarters of a pound of polar bear liver contains 7 or 8 *million* units of preformed vitamin A, this food is rightly forbidden by traditional Eskimo society. If it is of any satisfaction to you, polar bears themselves are at risk for vitamin A overdose since they routinely eat entire seals at one sitting. Seals, as we all know, are a very good source of vitamin A, yielding 30 to 100 million units per seal. Believe it or not, 6 million units of A have been taken by humans at once—in fact, five times in a row—without fatality. Naturally, this is idiotic, and especially so during pregnancy. Large prenatal doses of preformed oil (retinol) vitamin A can produce birth defects. However, deficiency of vitamin A also can, and it is much more likely. Human fetuses and newborn infants generally have low stores of vitamin A. Back in 1946, the AMA approved doses of 25,000 IU, but in the *Physicians' Desk Reference* you will find

cautions beginning at 6,000 IU during pregnancy. But it must be emphasized that this refers to the preformed, oil form of vitamin A, such as in fish oil or liver. These cautions do not apply to carotene, which the body only makes into vitamin A as it needs to. Occasional intake of large quantities of preformed vitamin A oil is probably quite safe during pregnancy, bearing in mind that a three-ounce serving of liver contains over 50,000 IU as retinol. I have yet to spot a pregnancy warning on supermarket packages of liver. Using carotene-rich green and orange vegetables and vegetable juices provides a vastly larger margin for error. These foods cannot possibly do any harm to mom or baby.

5. Take vitamin C. Because it is water-soluble, vitamin C is very safe at all times, including pregnancy. Frederick Klenner, M.D., gave large doses to three hundred pregnant women and reported virtually no complications in any of the pregnancies or deliveries. Indeed, the hospital nurses around Reidsville, N.C., noted that the infants who were healthiest and happiest were the "vitamin C babies." Other physicians have similarly reported that they have observed a complete absence of birth defects in babies born to vitamin C–taking mothers-to-be. Klenner gave 4,000 mg each day during the first trimester of pregnancy, 6,000 mg each day during the second trimester, and 10,000 mg each day during the third trimester. Klenner also gave booster injections of vitamin C to 80 percent of the women upon admission to the hospital for childbirth. The results? Wonderful, indeed: First, labor was shorter and sweeter. (My children's mother, with her three-hour and two-hour total labor times, can vouch for this.) Second, stretch marks were seldom seen. Third, there were no postpartum hemorrhages at all. Fourth, there were no toxic manifestations or cardiac distress. Fifth and most important, there were *no* miscarriages in the entire group of three hundred women.

Among Klenner's patients were the Fultz quintuplets, who at the time were the only quints in the Southeast to have survived. They were each given 50 mg of C daily at birth. This is an important point: if Mom is taking vitamin C, it has to be continued for *both* mother and baby afterward as well. Failure to do this will result in the well-publicized "rebound effect." Therefore, don't stop a good thing. If C is important enough for the woman to take before giving birth, then it is important enough for the baby to get after it has been born.

Varying amounts of vitamin C will be found in breast milk. If Mom takes a lot of C there will be C in the breast milk, too. If Mom is healing up and stressed out, there will probably be less C available to the baby. And if Mom is sick (or eating hospital food), there will almost certainly be a diminished C supply in her breast milk. The solution, again, is for both mother and baby to supplement with vitamin C.

We did exactly this with our babies, and were impressed with the results. You can finely powder a tasty chewable C tablet and put it on your finger or the baby's tongue. This should be done at every feeding. Infants do not need a lot of supplemental C, but they do need it frequently each day for maximum success. "Success" is easy to define: a healthy, happy baby that eats and sleeps well.

Very little vitamin C is found in formula, especially after it is packaged, opened, heated, poured, and oxidized during bottle feeding.

6. This is a tough order, but make time for your spouse so your baby will have two parents even after the novelty wears off. Fortunately, almost all authorities indicate that sex during pregnancy does not harm the baby. Common sense is needed, certainly, during the times immediately before and immediately after giving birth. But make a point to not neglect each other.

7. Avoid caffeine! It is America's most widely used and abused drug. Caffeine can enter the fetus's blood supply. Even two cups of coffee contains up to 250 mg of caffeine, a pharmacological dose. Five cans of cola have the same total amount, plus a lot more sugar (or, even worse, aspartame).

8. Concerned about high blood pressure? Then monitor your blood pressure, yourself, at home. It's easy and, because you avoid "white coat anxiety," it's actually more accurate than in a physician's office. You therefore reduce your chance of unneeded worry, unnecessary doctor interference, and resultant overprescription. If you are diagnosed with high blood pressure, consider taking a B-complex supplement before resorting to a drug. I know of a woman who was diagnosed with mild pre-eclampsia and chose to try a natural approach first. She took a B-complex tablet three to five times a day. She also cooked with the unfortunately-named "black fungus," a delicious mushroom found in many Oriental dishes. She used about two teaspoons of the dried mushroom, reconstituted in a cup of hot water before cooking, daily. Her blood pressure was normal in a few weeks. There were no further problems with the pregnancy.

9. Take vitamin E—at least 200 and perhaps 400 IU daily. This greatly reduces the chance of miscarriage. This is no myth: by the end of World War II, there were already dozens of medical studies confirming this. The cardiovascular benefits are excellent as well. Contrary to what many dieticians' textbooks say, getting foods containing other fat-soluble vitamins does NOT guarantee adequate vitamin E intake for pregnancy . . . or at any other time, for that matter.

10. Timing: age-wise, it is best to be pregnant when you are an adult woman. (Especially since adult men seem to have such trouble getting pregnant.) Better not to be an old woman or a girl. Risks to mother and child are greatly increased among very young and very old mothers. However, many of the risks are due to age-related nutritional deficits. A good diet, properly supplemented with folic acid (folate) and appropriate quantities of the other vitamins, will go a very long way to reduce birth defects.

Special Problems During Pregnancy and Lactation

Morning Sickness

1. Try a natural multivitamin, not an artificially colored one. Paint can be nauseating to eat.

2. Take all supplements on a full stomach, or better yet, in the middle of each meal.

3. Avoid ferrous sulfate iron supplements. Many doctors still prescribe this cookie-tossing form of iron in too large an amount, and without enough supplemental C for absorption. Constipation is almost guaranteed with ferrous sulfate. Use ferrous fumerate, ferrous gluconate, or especially carbonyl iron instead.

4. Try the homeopathic remedy Natrum Phos 6X for simple morning sickness, and possibly Kali Phos or Natrum Sulph.

5. You could also try some fresh, tasty juice first thing to get off to a good start in the morning. Fluids are always good, and it is a light, nutritious, natural way to get the blood sugar up.

6. Severe and prolonged vomiting requires medical attention.

Constipation

Constipation is quite common during gestation. It is also quite easy to avoid, as my charming chapter on hemorrhoids explains. Also, see the above recommendation about avoiding ferrous sulfate iron supplements. When pregnant, do not take medication for this or any other condition if you can possibly avoid doing so.

Weight Gain or Loss

Weight gain is natural, necessary, and desirable during pregnancy. A woman does *not* have to "get fat," however! My wife gained 25 pounds to deliver a 10 pound, 2 ounce baby girl. Though a slightly larger weight gain is normal and fine, it really should be no more than 35 pounds or so; under thirty is better. No fasting or weight loss attempts during pregnancy or lactation! Eat right and exercise appropriately, and the weight will take care of itself.

Hemorrhoids

Constipation can cause hemorrhoids, so see the constipation recommendations above. Also, avoid gulping unchewed cheese pizzas. Bear in mind that babies and amniotic fluid are heavy, which puts a lot of pressure on your rectum. Supplemental vitamin C will often help here, because C strengthens connective and vascular tissues. Topical application of vitamin E will also definitely help.

155

Heartburn

1. Eat frequent, small meals. In other words, "graze" rather than feast.

2. Chew your food especially well. This simple measure really works.

3. Combine your foods especially well. No need to obsess over this, but from your own experience, you can tell that some foods do not mix well in your stomach.

Recommended Reading

Bicknell F and Prescott F. *The Vitamins in Medicine,* 3rd edition. Milwaukee, WI: Lee Foundation, 1953.

Billings E and Westmore A. *The Billings Method.* New York: Ballantine, 1983.

Davis A. *Let's Eat Right to Keep Fit.* New York: Signet, 1970, 61.

Hillemann HH. *Developmental Malformation in Man and Other Animals.* [A Bibliography]. Milwaukee, WI: Lee Foundation, undated.

Hillemann HH. "Maternal Malnutrition and Fetal Prenatal Development Malformation" [Address at Oregon State College] (9 November 1956).

Hillemann HH. "Maternal Malnutrition and Congenital Deformity" [Address at Grants Pass, Oregon] (17 March 1958).

Hillemann HH. The spectrum of congenital defect, experimental and clinical. *Journal of Applied Nutrition* 14 (1961): 2.

Klein D. A coroner's-eye view of drug babies. *Los Angeles Times* (3 March 1991). [Cited in Farrell W. *The Myth of Male Power.* New York: Simon and Schuster, 1993, 413.]

Mendelsohn R. *Confessions of a Medical Heretic.* New York: Warner Books, 1979.

Mendelsohn R. *How to Raise a Healthy Child in Spite of Your Doctor.* Chicago: Contemporary Books, 1984.

Mendelsohn R. *Malepractice: How Doctors Manipulate Women.* Chicago: Contemporary Books, 1982.

Shute WE. *The Vitamin E Book.* New Canaan, CT: Keats Publishing, 1978.

Shute WE. *Your Child and Vitamin E.* New Canaan, CT: Keats Publishing, 1979.

Smith L, ed. *Clinical Guide to the Use of Vitamin C: The Clinical Experiences of Frederick R. Klenner, M.D.* Tacoma, WA: Life Sciences Press, 1988.

Stone I. *The Healing Factor.* New York: Grosset and Dunlap, 1972.

The Womanly Art of Breastfeeding, revised edition. Franklin Park, Illinois: La Leche League International, 1963.

Williams SR. "Nutrition During Lactation and Pregnancy" in *Nutrition and Diet Therapy,* 6th edition. St. Louis: Mosby, 1989.

At the time, I had never encountered a case of psoriasis before. So I looked it up in the *Merck Manual* while Frank sat there and waited as patiently as he could.

"It says here that there is no cure for psoriasis, Frank," I said hesitantly.

"That's what everybody has told me," he said. "But I think nutrition is worth a try."

I couldn't fault that reasoning.

"I've got to do something," Frank continued. "The doctors, and I've seen plenty of 'em, say there isn't anything they can do except give me these ointments and lotions. I said the ointments and lotions don't help. They said I should learn to live with it."

"How do you feel about that?" I asked.

"You can imagine how I feel!" Frank answered. "There is no way I'm going to spend the rest of my life itching and looking like this." Frank's psoriasis came and went periodically, but at that time it was back with a vengeance, and where the world could plainly see it: on his arms, neck, forehead, and face.

"What would you be willing to do to get well?" I responded.

"Anything," he said. "Anything at all, and I'm not kidding."

Frank was in his late twenties, energetic and prematurely bald. And resolute though he was, I expected that he was about to have his resolve sorely tested by what I suggested next: a complete change of diet to a naturopathic regimen of fresh foods and loads of vegetable juices, plus lecithin and assorted vitamins, including some extra vitamin D.

He didn't bat an eyelash.

I sensed that, unlike most people, Frank not only wanted it all but was willing to get his hands dirty to get it. He might, therefore, be willing to earnestly try the classic health-nut cure-all: fresh vegetable juice fasting. Really hard-core nature-cure quacks uniformly hold to the doctrine that whatever is wrong with a body, systemic toxemia is the root cause and fasting is the real cure. I presented the idea to Frank, who embraced it at once.

"So I could alternate a week of just vegetable juices with a week of a mostly fresh-and-raw diet," Frank concluded. I agreed. "How long do I keep it going? Oh, I know: until I'm symptom-free, of course."

"Provided you are feeling good doing it, yes."

So off he went to juice like crazy.

Right off the bat, Frank's psoriasis began to fade. He was much better within days. In little over a week, there was no trace whatsoever. But Frank's symptoms had gone away on their own before, so we all decided to bide our time.

Week after week, month after month, Frank stayed completely free of anything even remotely resembling psoriasis. He also felt better in unexpected ways: he said he was happier, sleeping better, thinking more clearly, had more energy, and hadn't a trace of a cold or any other sickness since he'd begun the program. He had lost a few pounds, but then his weight had leveled off automatically. He was one fit and trim, clear-skinned, happy guy.

Years passed, and Frank kept juicing on a regular basis. He never had psoriasis again. Of course, there is no cure for psoriasis, so this cannot be. Frank must have been deluded.

Yet I've seen this approach work on other people, too. Part-time vegetable juice fasting, employed intelligently, is safe and effective for reasonably healthy, nonpregnant people. Those who ridicule it should first meet Frank, who will confirm what it did for him.

Or his dermatologist, who now will, also.

Probably.

Rectal Bleeding

It's time to take the bull by the tail and face the situation.

W. C. FIELDS

Bleeding is scary, and rectal bleeding is the scariest. Margorie, age fifty-three, came to visit. She was losing half a cup of blood a day rectally. That is a lot of blood; a woman's entire five-day menstrual flow is only about that much in total. Marjorie was worried, and rightly so. She had seen an assortment of doctors and was currently under the care of a proctologist who could find nothing really wrong with her bowel. He found some slight, general inflammation during a sigmoidoscopy, but no lumps, bumps, polyps, or lesions of note. He told her that there was nothing to be done except keep an eye on it.

Keep looking. Not a nice thought under the circumstances.

Marjorie's question to me was the obvious one: what can be done? My standard answer, and it is also the truth, is that I wasn't sure, but natural therapies are generally worth a full and fair trial.

Years ago I had read an article from *California Medicine* about a doctor who treated bleeding peptic ulcers with cabbage juice, of all things. It was just crazy enough to get my attention: he gave one hundred hospitalized patients four glasses (yes, that's one full quart) of raw cabbage juice daily. The doctor, Garnett Cheney, M.D., reported pain relief in a few days, and healing in one third of the customary time. All this, not with medicines, not with surgery, but with cabbage juice. And he published his findings in a medical journal, no less. In 1953!

Figuring that it would be hard to hurt yourself with cabbages, unless you dropped them on your toe, I told Marjorie about the study. She was a lot more interested than a healthy person would have been, and said she'd do it. She had little to lose that she wasn't already losing.

Marjorie called back a week and a half later. She hadn't bought a juicer, but was putting fresh cabbage through her blender, and then straining it through cheesecloth to get the juice. She was drinking four glasses a day this way. Her bleeding had been reduced to a teaspoon on most days, and no blood at all on others. She was delighted. Then the really odd part of the conversation began: she had been to her proctologist, and told him of the improvement. He was pleased, of course; nothing odd about that. She then asked him if he'd care to know what she'd been doing lately. He said, certainly, he was a doctor, and was always interested to know what helps his patients. So she told him that she'd been drinking a quart of fresh, raw

159

cabbage juice every day. He stared back at her for a long moment, and then said, "No, that couldn't be it."

Marvel at this: to the specialist, it just couldn't have been due to the cabbage juice; it couldn't have been something that she had done on her own. Truth is, she got better in spite of him. He still got paid his specialist fees, of course.

Psychosis is spooky. Jim, a twenty-one-year-old, was brought to me by his mom and dad. They looked uncomfortable, and he looked miserable. Jim was a diagnosed schizophrenic. He was so violent that he had been—get this—kicked out of the state hospital and sent home to his parents. You've got to love that logic.

Jim had been completely unmanageable. He threatened his parents' lives on a daily basis and punched holes in the walls. He slept one hour per night, and roamed the city streets the other seven or eight. Jim is one of the premier reasons to not be out too late by yourself. His skin was scaly and his face severely broken out with acne. His dietary and digestive habits were appalling, and he was, to quote *Far Side* cartoonist Gary Larson, just plain nuts.

I faced this unhappy trio and felt helpless. The good part of it all was that they'd caught Jim on a good day (as far as I could see) and he wasn't going to tear up the place. From somewhere I recalled the three Ds of pellagra, that "extinct" niacin deficiency disease: dermatitis, dementia, and diarrhea. It was a reasonably close textbook match to the walking, talking Jim in front of me. I was also aware of the work of Abram Hoffer, M.D., a Canadian psychiatrist. Beginning in the early 1950s, Hoffer cured a vast number of psychotic patients with megadoses of niacin and vitamin C. The success of such vitamin treatments had earned him a quack's label too, of course.

But three feet away from me was a psycho with two terrified parents. Medical science had not helped him, and had, ironically, discharged him in the face of its own impotence. I told them about Dr. Hoffer's approach.

"We'll try anything," the father said, and the mother nodded energetically.

"Jim, how about you?" I asked.

"Yeah, I'll take the stuff," Jim said.

"I'll settle for that. Dr. Hoffer would have you take about 3,000 mg of niacin a day, and you'll want to take about 10,000 mg of vitamin C daily as well. Niacin deficiency actually causes psychosis, as well as the skin and GI problems that Jim happens to be experiencing. He may just need more niacin than the average person. Probably a lot more. At really large doses, niacin has a profound calming, sedating effect. Yet it is a nutrient, not a drug. The safety margin is huge. Dr. Hoffer has prescribed as much as 20,000 mg a day. 3,000 mg is not a particularly high dosage."

"And the vitamin C?" the father asked.

"Linus Pauling considered 10,000 mg for a man to be just an everyday dose," I answered. By body weight, it is about the same amount that a goat, cow, dog, cat, or rat would make each day. We cannot manufacture vitamin C because our livers lack a necessary enzyme, L-gulonolactone oxidase, and no, you cannot purchase and swallow that enzyme to do the job for you. Ask yourself: why would nature have these animals make that much for nothing? I think we should copy their example. These vitamins, at worst, are much less risky than any of the prescriptions Jim's ever tried."

Jim was silent and looked at his sneakers.

"How will we know if that's enough niacin?" his mother asked.

"If he behaves better, it's enough," I said. "If he takes too much niacin, he'll flush. That means his skin will get pink, or even red, especially the face, ears, and forearms. Sort of like a half-hour hot flash. You'll feel like you have a sunburn, Jim."

"That's okay with me," Jim said. "I like to be out at the beach."

They left, and I wondered how they'd managed to get by this far.

About two weeks later, Jim's father called for a follow-up conference. "Let me tell you what happened," he began. "You know Jim only sleeps maybe an hour a night? Well, the first night on the niacin, he slept eighteen hours. He's been sleeping about seven hours a night since."

"That's terrific," I said.

"That's not all," he said. "Last Friday morning, for the first time in I don't know how many years, Jim came down for breakfast. He walked into the dining room and said 'Good morning, Dad.'" Even on the phone I could hear the tears in the man's voice. It was wonderful.

There's more. Weeks later, Jim came in alone for an appointment. We sat down, and he told me that the niacin had worked, and that he'd stopped taking it.

"But why?" I asked. "It was helping you!"

"Yeah. Yeah. But I sort of like my sickness," Jim said.

I tried not to show my shock. This was nearly twenty years ago, and I hadn't yet learned that some psychotics simply prefer the psychotic state. As they get well, they may back away from the cure in favor of the disease.

Jim continued. "Whenever I get too far gone, though, I soak in a hot bath for a while and down a bottle of niacin. Then I feel fine." A whole bottle of niacin? That is literally what he said; I remember the line like it was uttered this morning. But if that's what he did, it seemed to work.

Here's the footnote: when a raving, dangerous patient can manage his illness and actually select the degree of psychosis he wants in his life, you have something unlike your standard idea of "cure." You have empowered a person to take responsibility for his life. And with the freedom that includes, you can get odd results.

Quick, how many psychoanalysts does it take to change a light bulb? One, but the light bulb has to really want to change.

Humor aside, we now are at a time when shrinks are breaking ranks. Some continue to say that the emotionally ill just need someone to talk to, to understand them and reason with them, but most want to drug patients into oblivion. Modern psychiatry has moved away from the Freudian couch and closer to Huxley's *Brave New World.* Prozac, Paxil, Zoloft, and their kin are our nonfictional soma, the mood-elevating wonder drugs that make psychoanalysis seem like the slow boat to China. Odd, really, that with a climate favoring medication over analysis, Abram Hoffer's niacin protocol is so unappreciated. After all, if "a gram is better than a damn," why not use grams of vitamins? Why not? Perhaps because niacin therapy is really, really cheap. There is no profit for the pharmaceutical companies, so why should the medical schools they fund teach upcoming doctors to use it?

Niacin, or vitamin B_3, has two forms: niacin and niacinamide. Both are water-soluble white powders. Your body obtains a small amount of niacin from metabolizing the essential amino acid tryptophan, found in protein. (60 mg of tryptophan yields about 1 mg of niacin).

Pellagra is the classic niacin-deficiency disease. It was once common in the rural South, where the poor had little else to eat except tryptophan-poor foods like milled corn. The symptoms are the three Ds I mentioned earlier: diarrhea, dermatitis, and dementia. More specific pellagra symptoms include weakness, anorexia, lassitude, indigestion, skin eruptions, skin scaling, neuritis, nervous system destruction, confusion, apathy, disorientation, and insanity.

Does this sound a bit like schizophrenia to you?

A few physicians thought so, too. They noticed that psychotics frequently had assorted pellagralike symptoms in addition to their mental problems. In the early 1950s, an insightful young psychiatrist named Abram Hoffer began clinical trials to see if there was a connection. He used very high doses of niacin, with very good results. He and his colleagues discovered that, whereas pellagra is a vitamin deficiency, schizophrenia is a vitamin dependency. For a while, niacin was used as a treatment for psychosis, but the convenience and relentless advertising of later "wonder drugs" diminished niacin's popularity. Then, the American Psychiatric Association unscientifically trashed megavitamin therapy in the 1970s. So now we have legions of nutritionally challenged, mentally-malnourished Americans who don't know it. And we pay out big bucks for behavior-modifying drugs that come factory-equipped with dangerous side effects.

Some additional and interesting therapeutic uses of niacin include Ménière's syndrome (chronic ringing in the ears plus nausea) and high-tone deafness. In long-term therapy, improvement was obtained with only 150–250 mg daily. Resistance to X-radiation was greatly improved at 500–600 mg daily. Nausea was also reduced. Supplemental niacin could therefore be of much value for cancer patients undergoing radiation therapy. Even healing after surgical shock and other trauma (such as burns, hemorrhage, and infection) is more rapid with niacin administration.

Niacin is very safe. "No toxicity has ever been shown for humans," Dr. Hoffer says. "For animals, it is about 6 grams per kilogram." This means that for an animal that weighs what a small human does (50 kg), a fatal dose would be some 300,000 mg, and nausea would prevent such a dose from being consumed long before this. The most

163

psychotic person you are ever likely to meet could probably not hold more than 15,000 mg per day, and most people, healthy or not, would never exceed a fraction of that. Physicians frequently give patients 2,000–5,000 mg of niacin to lower serum cholesterol. The safety margin is large. There is not even one death from niacin per year. The most common side effects of niacin therapy include flushing, skin itching, and, upon large overdose, nausea. Such symptoms vary with dose, the body's need, and volume of food consumed with the vitamin. I have noticed that taking large doses of vitamin C diminishes the side effects of very large doses of niacin. I think that patients should take at least twice as much C as niacin, and more C works even better.

Measurable niacin side effects, such as changes in liver function tests, tend to be a significant problem primarily in people with a history of alcohol abuse. But doctors citing such test variations as a reason why patients should not take megadoses of niacin are jumping to conclusions, Dr. Hoffer says. "Doctors confuse the elevation of liver function tests with underlying liver pathology, but this is wrong. It merely means that the liver is more active. And such changes can be prevented by taking some lecithin twice daily."

The real public health problem is a lack of niacin. The RDA is only about 20 mg. Half of all Americans will not get even that much from their diets. Niacin's special importance is indicated in that the RDA for niacin is twenty or more times higher than the RDA for other B vitamins, and that's just for everyday, healthy people.

Dr. Hoffer gave immensely higher doses, and it worked. I copied him with Jim, and that worked as much as Jim wanted it to. To continue your knowledge of niacin therapy, please see my chapter "Niacin Saturation" and consult the books found in the recommended reading for this chapter. I would actually go so far as to advise reading everything Dr. Hoffer has ever written.

Recommended Reading

Bicknell F and Prescott F. *The Vitamins in Medicine,* 3rd ed. Milwaukee, WI: Lee Foundation, 1953, 379.

Hawkins D and Pauling L. *Orthomolecular Psychiatry,* David Hawkins and Linus Pauling, eds., W. H. Freeman, San Francisco, 1973.

Hoffer A. *Hoffer's Law of Natural Nutrition.* Kingston, ON: Quarry Press, 1996.

Hoffer A. *Putting It All Together: The New Orthomolecular Nutrition.* New Canaan, CT: Keats Publishing, 1996.

Hoffer A. *Vitamin B$_3$ and Schizophrenia: Discovery, Recovery, Controversy.* Kingston, ON: Quarry Press, 1999.

Williams RJ, ed. *A Physician's Handbook on Orthomolecular Medicine.* New Canaan, CT: Keats Publishing, 1979.

Did you know that, according to the National Academy of Sciences, 8.5 million Americans take prescription sleeping pills at least once a year? Two million Americans take them every night for at least two months at a time! In addition to the inherent risks of sedative, hypnotic, or tranquilizing drugs, we are becoming a nation of nocturnal "users." With so many effective natural methods for falling asleep available, however, dependency on pharmaceuticals is completely unnecessary.

One of the best things about natural sleep aids is that they are safe and not habit forming. When your brain and body are well nourished, more restful sleep is a natural result. You are feeding your body, not drugging it. It is time for *everyone* to start saying no to excessively prescribed pharmaceuticals. Here are some techniques that will help you get to sleep more quickly and without drugs.

1. **Read** for a while. This will improve your mind while relaxing your body.

2. Get some **fresh air**. Open a window, walk the dog.

3. Try some moderate **exercise**, such as isometrics, yoga, or stretches. Couples have found that lovemaking works well, too. But you did not hear that from me.

4. Get more **L-tryptophan** in your diet. L-tryptophan is one of the amino acids your body uses to make serotonin and melatonin, neurotransmitters that help your brain to shut down for the night—and, therefore, be fully awake the next day. Seafood, milk, cheese, yogurt, and cashews are good sources of L-tryptophan. More of the L-tryptophan in dairy products gets to your brain when you have a carbohydrate along with it. That's why cheese and crackers, or milk and a whole-grain cookie, are good evening snacks. Normal portions can provide the target dose of about a gram (1,000 mg) or so. After all, a single portion (about a peanut-butter jar cap full) of cashews contains nearly 500 mg of tryptophan. Other nuts are almost as good, and seeds are even better. Chew them thoroughly, of course. That's half the fun of snacking, anyway, isn't it?

5. **Niacin** in larger than RDA doses will help induce sleep. Taking 50–200 mg about 20 minutes before bedtime usually works best. The amount required varies considerably from one person to another. Ideally, you take the least amount that makes you the most sleepy. Expect to experience a brief niacin "flush" (like a hot flash or blushing sensation), which is harmless and goes

away in short time. The warm feeling is pleasant to most people, but may be avoided by simply taking less niacin at any one time. A bit of practice will tell you how much you need. (See my chapter "Niacin Saturation.")

6. **Lecithin** makes up nearly a third of your brain's dry weight. This natural food substance is found in soy products and egg yolks and is available as a supplement as well. One or two tablespoons daily has consistently shortened the time needed for people to go to sleep.

7. **Meditation** may be very settling and help you sleep sooner and better. Certainly there are other benefits as well. The Transcendental Meditation technique has been shown to produce deep rest, reduced anxiety, and very effective relief from insomnia.

Ayurvedic Cycles

If you have tried all of the above and still find that you are one of those folks who fall asleep normally, but are wide awake at 3 A.M., and wonder what to do about it, I have an answer for you: get up. It may be perfectly normal for you to be awake then. Let's take a few moments to see what Ayurveda, India's great heritage of natural healing, counsels us when it comes to sleep. I am one of many people who, once able to unlearn some very Western assumptions of proper sleep habits, have found a natural fit with Ayurvedic cycles.

In Ayurveda there are three time periods in every twelve hours, called vata, pitta, and kapha. Vata is from 2–6, kapha is from 6–10, and pitta is from 10–2. The cycle repeats itself in the next twelve hours, so there are two vata times, two kapha times, and two pitta times each day. In a nutshell, Ayurvedic beliefs about sleep can be summed up, to borrow from Ben Franklin, as "Early to bed and early to rise makes a man healthy, wealthy, and wise."

During vata time, a person's mind is at its peak. Mental alertness is high, but so is a tendency toward mental excess, stress, and anxiety. Vata time is a good time to study, but a bad time to worry. It extends, remember, from 2–6 P.M. *and* 2–6 A.M. Without knowing about this, I, as a college student, used to do all my studying from when afternoon classes ended up until supper. My body was perhaps tired then, but my mind was fully on. Trappist monks start their day at about 2 A.M., promptly commencing with study until dawn. This too is an ayurvedic rhythm.

Pitta time, from 10–2, is a period of physical activity, appetite, and what we often call "getting our second wind." I know mothers and fathers who wait until the kids are in bed so they can get some work done. They tackle remodeling projects or clean the house starting at about 10 P.M. Once they get going, they can easily last until 2. Party-hearty college students are the ultimate pitta devotees. Their day is just beginning at 10 P.M., and goes great guns until 2 A.M.

If you want to stay awake, stay up for pitta time, but plan to be up for the whole

10–2 block. If you want to sleep, get to bed well before 10 P.M. This no doubt sounds unrealistically rigid to most people. That's too bad, because they are missing out on a good thing.

The good thing is kapha time, 6–10. Kapha is slow, smooth, easy, heavy . . . and sleepy. How do you feel after your evening dinner? Yeah, just kick back and put your feet up. Many of us doze off in the early evening. It is easy to do, because nature is trying to tell us something: go to bed, you lummox! And the earlier, the better.

And then there is morning kapha: 6 until 10. Sleepyheads everywhere know all about kapha time. When that alarm goes off at 6, and it's early, early dawn, and you cover your head with the pillow, or cuddle up with your blankets, sweetie, or Teddy bear, well, you know what I am talking about. Try to get a teenager up before 10. Not easy. Do you telephone your friends on weekends before 10 A.M.? Not if you want them to remain your friends.

When I was going through an unbelievably stressful period in my life, I could not sleep. No matter how tired I was, or how late I went to bed to get that tired, I would always wake up at the same time: very close to 2 or 2:30 A.M. This was driving me nuts, and in my desperation, I decided I had to try what you probably do not want to try: going to bed really early (again, like the Trappists do), around 8 P.M. I was surprised that I fell asleep so readily. I still woke up at 2, but by then I'd had six hours of sleep. With time, I was able to "sleep in" until 4 A.M. My life stresses were unabated, but I had a reliable eight hours of sleep each night with which to attack them. Sounds odd, of course, but it works.

Recommended Reading

Chopra D. *Perfect Health.* New York: Harmony Books, 1991.

Lad V. *Ayurveda: The Science of Self-Healing.* Santa Fe, NM: Lotus, 1984.

There is a nutritional alternative for most drugs. You have to dig a bit for the details, but the work has been done. You will find very few negative effects from vitamins in the *Physicians' Desk Reference* (*PDR*), but you will see column after column and page after page of side effects, contraindications, and warnings for drugs.

For example, I give you Coumadin, the ubiquitous drug for thinning the blood. You can often use vitamin E instead. Vitamin E potentiates the effects of Coumadin, and at up to 3,200 IU or less daily, it can completely and safely substitute for the drug. That is just plain true. I've seen it again and again.

The case of the Big Trucker stands out in particular.

Bob was a big guy: tall, wide, and heavy. He had a lengthy history of thrombophlebitis and most of its possible complications. One day he came to see me, wondering what options he had to forever taking Coumadin.

"You need to lose weight, Bob," was the first thing I said. "You need to stop smoking, too. There's no way any therapy, drug, or anything else is going to really work for you unless you do those things first."

He listened thoughtfully. "OK," he said. "I'll try. What else?"

Pleased that we'd even gotten this far without his wiping the floor with me, I proceeded to tell this man of few words about vitamin E as a blood thinner. Doctors Wilfrid Shute and Evan Shute of London, Ontario pioneered such use of the vitamin back in the 1940s. Their medical society went berserk, blacklisted them from meetings, and expelled any doctor that even attended a lecture by the Shute brothers.

Vitamin E is vastly safer than warfarin, the generic name of Coumadin. Warfarin is the active ingredient in rat poison. Rats are pretty smart, by the way. They must be poisoned subtly and long-term, like patients. A cumulative moderate overdose of Coumadin causes their blood to be too thin, and the little bastards hemorrhage and die. A cumulative overdose of vitamin E, even extreme megadosing, has never killed anybody.

Bob's prothrombin (clotting) time was 13 seconds without medication. His doc wanted 20–22 seconds, and got it with the drug. "Will I get the same results with vitamin E?" Bob asked.

"You might," I said. "Ask your doctor to try a gradual reduction dosage of the drug while gradually increasing the vitamin dosage. I've seen that work well before."

Weeks later I saw Big Bob again. He had stopped smoking and lost weight.

"How are you doing?" I asked him leadingly.

"Pretty good," Bob admitted. "Still on the Coumadin. Not taking the vitamin E yet."

"Why?" I asked.

The answer really surprised me.

"Well," Bob said, "I really don't want to talk to the doctor about it. He'll think I'm stupid. Says I've got to take it."

"You feel you can't talk to your doctor about this?"

"Nope. I didn't even finish high school," Bob said. "He'll just make me feel like a jerk for wanting to not take my medicine."

Witnessing a big, strong man shrink childishly away from confronting his own doctor was a new one for me. "You can talk to your doctor, Bob. You've got to be able to discuss your own body with your doctor. What did he say to you when he observed that you'd lost weight?"

"He said just keep doing what I'm doing."

"And stopping the smoking?" I added.

"He said that was good, too," Bob answered. "He never brought that up before, but he said it was good that I'd quit." Incredibly, the great majority of patients who smoke have never been ordered to quit by their doctor.

"But our credit isn't good enough for vitamin E, huh?" I said with a half smile. "You know, you're not offering anything foolish when you ask for a tapering drug dosage schedule and willingly come in for regular monitoring. The safer alternative is always worth a therapeutic trial; any doctor should know that."

Bob shook his head. He paused, then shook it again. "No," he said. "Don't want to bring it up with him." There was a pause. "I'm just going to take the vitamin E anyway," Bob said quietly.

"I'd prefer the doctor was in on this," I responded, "but if you are going to do it, do it right. Increase the dose over a period of weeks. Most people start with 200 IU daily, and eventually get to between 1,200 and 2,400 IU daily. Do it gradually, and here's a way to tell how you're coming: go in to your doctor regularly, as you always do. Have him check your protime, as he always does. If you get the numbers he wants, he won't care how you got them."

"Could I increase the vitamin E and still stay on the Coumadin?" Bob wondered.

"More or less, but the more E you take, the stronger the Coumadin's effect. You'll probably get to the point where your protime is too long, and he'll have to cut back on the dosage of Coumadin."

Bob thought about that for a bit. "So I can just show him that I don't need the drug any more?"

"That's about it," I said. "If your protime is on the long side, he'll cut you back on the medicine."

A month later I saw Bob for a follow-up visit. "I did it," he said. "The last time I saw the doctor, my clotting time was a bit too long. So he asked me, 'What are you doing?' I

169

told him I was taking vitamin E. He said, 'Stop taking that vitamin. It is interfering with the Coumadin.' "

Golly, Doc, we wouldn't want that, now would we?

Thanks to the J.J. Newberry department store, I avoided hand surgery. Twice. Newberry's, in Batavia, New York, was a creaky, wooden-floored, iron-ceilinged five-and-dime. From the worn chrome lunch counter, selling hot dogs basted in grease, to the claustrophobic basement, where they kept the pet department (and the iguanas), every trip to Newberry's was a trip back into the forties. Friends and I made a pilgrimage to the store every time we were in town.

I'd been having some trouble with my left hand. A chiropractor friend of mine told me I was developing a trigger finger, and he sure had that right. Whenever I curled my hand, my ring finger locked in the down position. This was especially disturbing to me because both my mother and father had surgery for trigger fingers—in Dad's case, nine such operations! Oh, great, I thought. My turn now, at age thirty, in graduate school.

One evening, there I was in statistics class, trying to stay awake. My hand was aching and locking so that I wiggled and squirmed constantly. Class members probably thought I had to go to the bathroom. I flexed my hand, stretching and curling it. I cracked my knuckles (silently) and bent my wrist. Hmm. It all felt a bit better, but nothing remarkable. This impromptu experimentation went on sporadically, stimulated by the dullness of standard deviations, two-tailed t-tests, and chi squares.

Then I grabbed my wrist with my other hand, and applied some downward traction. I felt a pull, then a clunk, in my wrist. I grabbed a thicker part of my arm, closed my hand and curled my fingers around it and pulled, and it happened again. By then I'd nearly lost track of the lecture, just like everybody else had, but for a different reason. I left off my experimenting and hastened back to note-taking and question-asking.

So back to Newberry's, the five-and-dime, remember? It was a Friday evening, about 5:30. I was squeaking my way around the store, bargain hunting. Down one war-torn, metal-shelved isle, I spotted some three-inch diameter hard rubber balls. They were probably designed for playing fetch with your favorite medium-sized dog. They were solid rubber, unpainted, and three for a dollar. I summoned up unknown instincts, took the plunge, and bought two.

I still had the trigger finger problem. But I had pocketed the experience from statistics class that grabbing something, curling my hand, and stretching my wrists got me a clunk in the wrist and some relief. Holding one of the balls in my hand, I began to do the same procedure. I found that if I grabbed the ball with my fingers only (no thumb), I could roll the ball from fingertips to wrist, bending my hand more and more as I went. Furthermore, if I braced my wrist with the other hand, I could choose where the hand and wrist actually bent and stretched the most. The tangible rewards were straightforward: a clunk in the wrist and profound relief in the hand.

There are over fifty bones between your two hands. That's about one quarter of all the bones in your body. Your wrist is made up of many small bones through which a complicated robotic system of nerves, blood vessels, ligaments, and tendons must pass. The idea of physiotherapy for carpal tunnel syndrome and other repetitive motion disorders is hardly new, but this "hardball" approach for trigger fingers was never offered to anyone I've met.

Bottom line was that it was completely successful. Over a period of three weeks at most, all the triggering went away. No pain, soreness, or stiffness. No locking. Just a 34 cent (plus tax) ball from Newberry's, used a couple of times a day.

Newberry's has since gone out of business, but there's more. During my once-a-decade physical, I asked my doctor about a lump on my wrist. It was small and hard, on the outside wrist two inches south of my thumb.

"Ganglionic cyst," he said.

Ah yes, the "Bible" cyst. In the old days, doctors just whacked them out of existence with whatever big book was at hand. This guy referred me to a hand specialist instead.

The hand surgeon explained to me how he would set out my arm like this, use an anesthetic like so, cut off the blood supply here, and open an incision there. More details followed, which made me squeamish.

"What will happen if I don't choose to have the surgery?" I asked.

"It might get worse; it probably won't get better," he answered.

I was instructed to stop and schedule a date for surgery on my way out with one of a pack of office assistants, but I kept right on walking. I wasn't sure I wanted to go through all of that for a wrist lump.

I continued to use my exercise ball a few times a week to keep any chance of the trigger finger from returning.

Time passed.

One day I noticed that the wrist lump was gone. Nobody hit me with the Old Testament, and nobody operated, either. The lump has never returned, no it never returned, and its fate is still unlearned.

Newberry's saved my insurance company a pile of money, saved me two surgeries, and I get to keep the balls. Total cost of my therapy: 67 cents.

Plus tax.

Vaccinations

uch of what I've shared with you throughout this book might be regarded as good common sense, and a rapidly increasing number of parents share the "vitamins yes, junk food no" point of view. Now for the really controversial part: my children did not get immunizations. My boy had two rounds of shots as an infant, but when his mother and I both saw that the vaccinations made him sick, we halted them. A lot of eyebrows may raise at this point, and that's fine. Let's raise them a bit further.

Criticism of vaccinations is by no means a new phenomenon. Some fifty years ago, William McCormick, M.D., of Toronto, published a series of papers (please see the Bibliography for an extensive list of McCormick's work) showing that inoculations have had very little, if any, influence on the history of these illnesses. In 1960, Howard H. Hillemann's lengthy paper, "The Illusion of American Health and Longevity," presented similar findings. Pediatrician Robert Mendelsohn was an outspoken critic of vaccination throughout the 1970s and 1980s. The debate continues to this day, with the Internet providing one of the major forums for discussion. (See the end of this chapter for websites.) So before your heart stops at the thought of my meatless, shotless children, read these researchers' papers and start wondering not why my kids aren't "protected" but if yours really are. If you're a young parent with young children, the question of vaccinations for your family is an important one. You want what's best for your kids. We all do. So what's the right decision, then? Shots or no shots?

There is plentiful evidence that vaccinations are less than beneficial. The venerable British Anti-Vaccination League (and, incidentally, George Bernard Shaw) were vociferously against them. Homeopathic medical writers frequently include passages in their texts on how to treat vaccinosis, or the side effects of vaccinations.

Certainly the U.S. government cannot say without qualification that shots are either safe or essential. After all, this is what was said about the infamous swine flu vaccine in a 1976 FDA consumer memo: "Some minor side effects— tenderness in the arm, low fever, tiredness—will occur in less than 4 percent of [vaccinated] adults. Serious reactions from flu vaccines are very rare." So much for blanket claims of safety, for many persons well remember the numerous and serious side effects of swine flu vaccine that forced the federal immunization program to a halt.

As far as being essential, in the same memo the FDA said this of the vaccine: "Question: What can be done to prevent an epidemic? Answer: The only preventive action we can take is to develop a vaccine to immunize the public against the virus. This will prevent the virus from spreading." This was seen to be totally false. After all, the public immunization program was abruptly halted and still there was no epidemic of swine flu.

Surely there are other factors involved in prevention of illness or epidemic. But try telling that to allopathically oriented health commissioners and doctors. You'd think that monks and nuns who work with the sick would get all their patients' diseases . . . but they seldom do. There is much more to wellness than just collecting shots. Real wellness is the result of healthful living: natural diet, whole raw foods, plentiful vitamins, internal cleansing through periodic juice fasting, ample rest, peace of mind, and appropriate confidence in Nature's preference to keep us alive and well. If we follow these parameters, the essence of naturopathy, we find inoculations to be irrelevant.

Now if you live on candy, hamburgers, shakes, and steaks, you'd best get inoculated. Just as overfed, undernourished laboratory rats get sick at any brush with disease, so do overfed, undernourished people. A weakened, polluted body is fertile ground for assorted microbes to multiply. To the extent that vaccines and drugs deal with microbes only, they are apparently effective.

That phrase was "apparently" effective. Like adding Drano to a polluted pond, the chemical intervention does produce some dead germs. But poison on top of poison fails to get at a root cause of all illness, which is "polluted body" or systemic toxemia. In fact, the added drugs and vaccines compound the body's problem, for they cause side effects and new troubles of their own. The person gets more vaccines and still more drugs, to try to cover all these new illnesses, and then even more illness results. The cycle can go on and on for a lifetime, never solving the real problem.

Body pollution from wrong diet and neglect of natural living principles causes disease. How can inoculations be given for neglect? How can you vaccinate a body against abuse? How can you be immunized against bad diet and insufficient vitamins? It can't be done. The allopathic medical establishment is looking into test tubes for answers that are found at our dinner tables. Drug companies' chemicals and hospitals' equipment cannot eliminate disease because they do not bring health in its place. Only you, yourself, can live in such a way as to become and stay well. Then the underlying causes of illness, including those we're usually immunized against, are eliminated without vaccination.

This applies to children, as well as to adults. If children are fed vitamin-rich, raw and whole food diets, they will not require shots to stay healthy. They will be healthier without the vaccination. We would do well to remember the examples of the Hunza (in Pakistan) and other truly isolated "primitive" peoples who are so healthy they don't even have names for diseases that we're seeking immunizations for. They have no shots, no free clinics, and no filled-in vaccination charts—until they start eating "civilized man's" foods. When they start into a diet of processed foods, sugar, and white flour and rice, they promptly contract all the "infectious" diseases.

There is proof. Years ago, Weston Price, a dentist, went around the world to observe

174

primitive peoples and their diet. He found that a simple, natural diet of mostly raw and always whole foods was the common denominator among all healthy, disease-free primitive peoples. Once these peoples started developing a Western diet, however, cavities began to appear, along with tuberculosis, pneumonia, influenza, and other diseases.

There are alternatives to having one's children routinely vaccinated. There is the choice of simply not having shots. No one should order you to get shots for your kids or order you not to get them. A lot of people may try, however. I believe that the parents should decide. Many parents, including my wife and me, have chosen to decline vaccinations for their children after careful deliberation. In doing so, we sometimes run into not unexpected opposition for this decision. Among the arguments you're likely to hear against no-shots policies (all false) are:

1. You don't care about your kid's health. You're only thinking of your own ideologies.

2. Vaccination is legally required. You must have it done or your kids can't go to school.

3. Kids will get the diseases unless they're immunized against them.

4. You're taking a chance. Why not get the shots and be safe?

Let's consider each of these arguments in turn.

Argument 1: You Don't Care

The truth is, we really do care about our children and their health, and that is the number one reason why they are not getting inoculations. We don't want to inject unnecessary poisons into our children. We want our kids to be down deep, totally healthy. A well-nourished, near-vegetarian, no-drug, vitamin-supplemented child is a truly healthy child. We care for our children very, very much, as the vast majority of parents do.

Argument 2: It's the Law

Vaccination is not legally required. For entrance into public schools, yes, shots are normally required. For certain jobs, yes again. Naturally the military requires them. There are ways of getting around these individual regulations, though. The simplest way is to take religious exception to vaccination on personal, moral, and spiritual grounds. This is constitutionally valid; remember that the First Amendment guarantees freedom of religion. There are two religious avenues to consider, and we have used them both.

Church Membership

First, you can join a religious group that holds vaccinations in disfavor. If this is unacceptable or impractical, you can start a church organization that believes vaccinations are morally wrong. You can create a bona fide religious organization by first becoming a legally ordained minister through the mail for $25 or so from various churches. I do not assert that by-mail ordinations put you on a par with the Pope; I merely assert that they are legal. With such an ordination you can start your own religious group with your own set of doctrinal beliefs. These beliefs may certainly "forbid any serum, vaccine, foreign, unnatural, or chemical substance of any nature to be injected or ingested into a church member's body for any avowed medical purpose whatsoever."

Personal Religious Belief

The second variant depends on your state's laws. Some states (such as New York, where I live) no longer require a designated church affiliation because to do so would probably be unconstitutional. Instead, parents or guardians must hold genuine and sincere religious beliefs that are contrary to vaccinations. This means that a simple affidavit stating those beliefs in one or two sentences may suffice. An affidavit is as simple as having both parents sign their two-sentence statement in the presence of a notary public. The notary will then stamp the paper, which instantly becomes a rather powerful document. Your bank or town clerk will likely notarize for little or no charge. What does such a vaccination exemption letter look like? Well, it might look a lot like the one my children used:

It is my sincerely held religious belief that immunization is detrimental to the health and purity of the body, mind, and spirit. Therefore, I respectfully request that my child,

_____, *be allowed to attend school, namely*
(student's full name here)

_____, *without being immunized.*
(school's full name and address here)

_____   _____
Mother's signature   Father's signature

Sworn to before me this _____ *th day of* _____, 20_____.

_____
Notary Public

It has always been relatively simple for well-informed, determined parents to have their children attend school without any shots if they choose a religious exemption. But what about parents of children who are already partially immunized, who change their mind? They have often been denied a religious exemption due to health department or school officials' claims that their religious beliefs are not "sincerely held" since they have already had vaccinations prior to their new request for religious exemption. In January 2002, however, U.S. District Court Judge Michael Telesca wrote an important precedent-setting decision: "This court may not pass on the wisdom of belief, nor on the manner upon which she came to hold that belief, provided that she maintains a sincere and genuine religious objection to immunization." In other words, once a person decides, for reasons of religious conscience, that she does not want any more shots, her decision is valid even if she previously had her child immunized. The case is also important because the family in question was devoutly Roman Catholic. The Vatican is not opposed to vaccination. This decision allows individual members of a mainstream church organization to hold personal spiritual beliefs that conflict with their church's official doctrine.

Medical Exemption

A completely different way to get around a vaccination requirement is to prove to a medical doctor that your children would suffer a great health risk by being vaccinated. A possible allergic reaction to the shot(s) would be an ideal reason, although great susceptibility to side effects or a pre-existing high-risk condition could also be given as reasons. This is hard to do; most physicians will side with orthodoxy and public health policy, because if not, they might be called on the carpet by authorities to defend why they think a child shouldn't be vaccinated. This approach, then, puts burden of proof on both you and the doctor, and will only be as strong as the weaker link.

Alternative Education

Still another way to avoid shots for kids might be to enroll them in a private, cooperative, or alternative school that does not discriminate on medical grounds. It might be possible for a group of concerned parents to create such a school to ensure freedom of choice for family health decisions. However, most private and parochial schools are subject to, and in enthusiastic compliance with, the same public health regulations as public schools.

Home schooling is certainly an option. There are families in your community who teach their own children at home, and there are state education requirements that they must meet to do so. There are no inoculation requirements, however. You can keep the government happy and your kids' minds open at the same time by home schooling. Warning: it is labor intensive, to be sure.

Argument 3: Unvaccinated Kids Are Sitting Ducks

Kids don't automatically "get" all those so-called diseases of childhood. Just as insects eat weak crops, disease thrives in weak bodies. As I've said in this chapter, and as observations of primitive societies have shown, healthy lifestyles and diets are enough to prevent most of the diseases of modern society. My kids stay healthy not because of injections but because of correct eating and naturally strengthened immune systems.

Argument 4: Just in Case, To Be Safe

Not getting vaccinations may actually be safer than getting them. Consider the DPT shot. Hundreds of millions of dollars have been paid out to parents of vaccine-disabled or vaccine-killed children. According to statistics compiled by the National Vaccine

Information Center, between July 1990 and November 1993 "1,576 children died from adverse reactions to common vaccines" in the United States. That works out to 38 per month. Most deaths were from the pertussis (whooping cough) vaccine. In unimmunized Great Britain, in 1978 and 1979 there were 36 deaths attributed to whooping cough itself. Even allowing for wide variation in sample dates and population, it is impossible to dismiss the fact that *more American kids died from shots in a month than British kids died without shots in two years.*

Readers should also keep in mind that careful study of the medical profession's own statistics fails to verify the very common and highly emotional viewpoint that vaccination has been the major factor in the reduction of infectious diseases. Reviews of the medical literature show that the dramatic decline in typhoid, diphtheria, and whooping cough in this country occurred *before* vaccinations were available. Even polio fatalities decreased by nearly 90 percent from 1915 to 1955, before the polio vaccine became available. How can we truly say, then, that vaccination was the key factor? There was a medical doctor in Canada who treated polio with iodine supplements in the 1950s. The effectiveness of his treatments suggests that the popularization of iodized salt has had more to do with the elimination of polio than has the polio vaccine!

Now I am not saying that there's no value to the Salk vaccine. But I do think that a vegetarian diet, a little iodine, and a lot of vitamin C will actually prevent polio more effectively. Much support for a shot-free lifestyle can be found in articles available in *Mothering* magazine, from the National Vaccination Information Center, or on the Internet. You will especially want to know of a series of papers on using vitamin C to inactivate polio viruses, written by D. C. Jungeblut in the 1930s.

Why face side effects, contraindications, reactions, and added toxins, especially when there is poor evidence for vaccines' efficacy? How is that being safe?

It is not enough to just say "no" to shots. You have to take active, alternative measures to protect your children's health in their stead. There is a strong track record for preventing diseases through really good nutrition. My children were raised virtually vegetarian, and I say again that vegetarians statistically are less subject to infectious illness. When they were preschoolers, my children received 250–500 mg of vitamin C with each meal. As they got older, they got more C. In my opinion, a good prevention plan is to give kids half their age in grams of C per day. That means that an eight-year-old would get 4,000 mg per day and a twelve-year-old would get 6,000 mg per day, and so forth. (Always divide up the doses.) These are everyday health maintenance amounts. If you think they are too high, it is high time to read more on the subject in this book, and read more books on the subject as well. The bibliography is a good starting place for skeptics and their physicians.

It is vital (and also comforting) to remember that vitamin C is a proven antibiotic, antitoxin, and antiviral. (*The Healing Factor,* by Irwin Stone, discusses this in detail.) When my children had a fever or cough, they were put to bed with a temporarily all-fruit or vegetable-juice diet, saturation levels of vitamin C, and required to rest. They got better. And, although unvaccinated, they have never had whooping cough, polio, diphtheria, or measles. Was it just dumb luck, or was it smart eating?

Although I have offered my family's personal vaccination viewpoint to the reader, I do not pretend to tell anyone to get shots or not to get shots. Parents must make their own decisions based on all the facts they can gather. To assist in this search, I suggest reading the books by Robert Mendelsohn listed in the Recommended Reading, as well as *A Shot in the Dark* by Harris Coulter and Barbara Fisher, which focuses on the pertussis vaccine. I most earnestly recommend *Vaccinations: The Rest of the Story,* and a good Internet search.

Recommended Websites

- www.vaccinationnews.com
- www.thinktwice.com
- www.vaccines.bizland.com
- www.avn.org.au
- www.909shot.com
- www.redflagsweekly.com
- www.vaccination.inoz.com

Recommended Reading

Coulter HL and Fisher BL. *A Shot in the Dark.* Garden City Park, NY: Avery, 1991.

Edward JF. Iodine: its use in the treatment and prevention of poliomyelitis and allied diseases. *Manitoba Medical Review* 34 (1954): 337–39.

Hillemann HH. The illusion of American health and longevity. *Clinical Physiology* 2 (1960): 120–77.

Jungeblut CW. Inactivation of poliomyelitis virus by crystallin vitamin C (ascorbic acid). *Journal of Experimental Medicine* 62 (1935): 517–21.

Jungeblut CW. Further observations on vitamin C therapy in experimental poliomyelitis. *Journal of Experimental Medicine* 65 (1939): 127–46.

Jungeblut CW. A further contribution to the vitamin C therapy in experimental poliomyelitis. *Journal of Experimental Medicine* 70 (1939): 327–46.

Mendelsohn RS. *Confessions of a Medical Heretic.* Chicago: Contemporary Books, 1979.

Mendelsohn RS. *How to Raise a Healthy Child in Spite of Your Doctor.* New York: Ballantine Books, 1985.

Mothering Magazine. *Vaccinations: The Rest of the Story.* Chicago: Mothering Books, 1993.

Price WA. *Nutrition and Physical Degeneration.* La Mesa, CA: Price-Pottenger Nutrition Foundation, 1945, revised 1970.

Smith L, ed. *Clinical Guide to the Use of Vitamin C: The Clinical Experiences of Frederick R. Klenner, M.D.* Tacoma, WA: Life Sciences Press, 1988.

Tokasz J. Judge forces school to accept girl. Rochester, NY: *Democrat and Chronicle* (31 Jan 2002), B-1.

Part Two

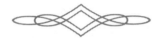

Natural Healing Tools and Techniques

Saul's Super Remedy

The physician should not treat the disease,
but the patient who is suffering from it.
MAIMONIDES

"Why, it's good for what ails you." That's how my great-uncle described the virtues of any food or edible plant he knew to be healthy. Quite a few made his list, and as a result, I disliked nearly everything he put on the dinner table when we came to visit. But I always remembered this saying of his, along with his standard greeting when he met us at his front door: "Come in, and make your miserable lives happy!"

Recently, a lady wrote to me wanting a cure for eczema. I get a lot of letters like that, all of which I answer with a suggestion to do some reading. Not everybody likes a response like that. I mentioned that she could do a site search at DoctorYourself.com, using the keyword "skin" as a starting point. That will bring up seventy-four matches. She replied that that was too general to really help her, for she wanted a specific cure for eczema.

And therein lies the problem.

Most folks want to know how to treat a particular disease condition, but are not interested in how to treat their whole body. Yet, you cannot remove the first from the second. It sounds like a truism, but the way to get rid of a skin disease is to have healthy skin. Treating symptoms is allopathy (drug medicine). Natural healing is about treating the person with the symptoms. The quote at the beginning of this chapter is a good reminder for all of us. "Holistic" is more than a philosophy or catchy title. It is a way of life that is "good for what ails you." You can exclude illness by actively creating a healthy body every day.

As you've probably already noticed, I advocate megadoses of vitamins (generally in conjunction with exercise, good diet, and stress reduction) for a wide array of different health conditions. Is this because I'm a simpleton obsessed with vitamins? No, it's because what we call diseases are usually just different manifestations of the same problem: the huge vitamin deficiencies most of us silently and chronically endure. Get rid of the deficiency, and the disease disappears.

LAW: The quantity of a nutritional supplement that cures an illness indicates the patient's degree of deficiency. It is therefore not a megadose of the vitamin, but rather a megadeficiency of the nutrient that we are dealing with.

Doctors would like you to believe that your health is very complicated, with thousands of diseases out there requiring thousands of patented drugs and trained experts to figure out what to use to keep you upright. But the truth is, health is pretty simple. The body evolved to last a long lifetime on only about two dozen naturally occurring nutrients. None of the basic building blocks of life are pharmaceutical drugs, not one. All living things in creation owe their lives to nature, not to technology. Live right and medical intervention should play only a tiny role in your life.

In that spirit, I offer you my special do-it-yourself super remedy. If you do not feel well—and I would go so far to say for almost any reason—try this deceptively simple game plan. Go out of your way to promptly get to saturation of the following four key nutrients: niacin, vitamin C, water, and carotene. Then cut the junk out of your diet. This plan is uncomplicated, fast-acting, and very effective on a wide variety of illnesses. Elsewhere in the book I offer megadosing routines customized to a particular condition, but often I just refer you back to this one, because so many diseases are caused by a need for these four nutrients. If in doubt, this is the place to start.

1. **Get to niacin saturation**, which is indicated by a mild, warm, pink-eared facial vasodilation known as a "flush." (Inside Windsor Castle it is doubtless known as a "royal flush.") If you are feeling stressed, anxious, depressed, worried, or just plain ticked off, try this while you are pouring that double shot of bourbon and counting to ten: immediately take 50 to 100 mg of niacin (not niacinamide) every ten minutes until you feel nice and toasty. . . and happy. Then continue to take enough niacin throughout the day so that each dose makes you feel just a tad warm. If you think this will not work, it's because you have not tried it. I refer to the niacin, not the bourbon.

   While we're at it, some Fearless Flush Facts: If I had a dime for every person worried about the flushing they experienced when taking large doses of niacin, I'd be a rich man. Niacin flushes are harmless. Some people (including me) enjoy them, especially in winter, as they are accompanied by some welcome warmth. Dr. Abram Hoffer says that the more niacin you take now, the less you will flush later. (See my chapter "Niacin Saturation" for more information.)

   Time needed to see improvement: less than an hour.

2. **Get to vitamin C saturation**, which is indicated by bowel tolerance. That means take a few thousand mg of vitamin C every ten minutes until you get, or feel like you are about to get, diarrhea. When you feel a rumbling in the bowel, you are close to bowel tolerance and can slightly reduce the amount of C that you've been taking. As you get well, you will find that the amount of C your body can hold automatically goes down. Follow my "Take enough C to be symptom free" rule. This will both

clean you out and jump-start your immune system. Vitamin C in quantity is the best broad-spectrum antitoxin, antibiotic, and antiviral there is. Cheapest, too. See my chapter "Vitamin C Megadose Therapy" for more information.

Time needed to see improvement: less than a day.

3. **Get to carotene (and water) saturation.** These can be simultaneously achieved by twice daily juicing a big stack of green or orange vegetables, such as carrots. Yes, green, as well as orange, veggies are absolutely loaded with carotene. Yes, you really do have to drink it. What are you afraid of? When's the last time a person died of vegetable overdose?

Saturation of carotene is reached when your skin turns a partial pumpkin color. Called "hypercarotenosis," it is harmless. Looks cool, too, much like a suntan.

Abundant water intake is guaranteed by abundant juicing. When your tummy is full of juice, you will need to urinate a lot. That is all I mean by water saturation. Inside your skin, you are an aquatic animal. Water is good. Veggie juice is better. If you are worried about getting enough trace minerals, relax: most are amply found in the vegetables. See my chapter "Juicing" for more information.

Time needed to see improvement: less than a week.

Commonsense caution: If your doctor has instructed you to limit fluids, then do so. Instead of juicing, you can eat Blender Salads for easy-to-assimilate raw veggie power. A recipe is provided in my chapter "Kidney Disease."

4. **Stop eating meat, sugar, and chemical food additives.** Be a vegetarian, or at least come as close as you can. There is nothing to it; just eat the other, good natural foods that you really like anyway—salads, nuts, your favorite vegetables, brown rice and other whole grains, fruits, and beans. Buy fresh or read every label. No chemicals, no sugar. Just do it!

Time needed to see improvement: less than two weeks.

If you think I've lost what's left of my marbles, think again. I have never been more serious. When I work with very sick people, the first "homework" I give them is to go flush, reach bowel tolerance, hydrate, turn orange, and save a cow. Sounds preposterous, doesn't it? But people who do so feel better immediately. Their tests improve immediately. And they learn something of lasting practical value.

Niacin Saturation

Niacin is vitamin B_3, one of the water-soluble B-complex vitamins. One of its unique properties is its ability to help you relax and get to sleep at night. In quantity, it is a superb antipsychotic. And it is well established that niacin helps reduce harmful cholesterol levels in the bloodstream.

Niacin has the ability to reduce anxiety and relieve depression. Yet another feature of niacin is that it dilates blood vessels and creates a sensation of warmth, called a "niacin flush." This is often accompanied with a blushing of the skin. It is this flush, or sensation of heat, that indicates a temporary saturation of niacin, and that is our topic here.

The Niacin Flush

When you flush, you can literally see and feel that you've taken enough niacin. The idea is to initially take just enough niacin to have a slight flush. This means a pinkness about the cheeks, ears, neck, forearms—and perhaps elsewhere. A niacin flush should end in about ten minutes or so. If you take too much niacin, the flush may be more pronounced and longer lasting. If you flush beet red for half an hour and feel weird, well, you took too much. As large doses of niacin on an empty stomach are certain to cause profound flushing, take your niacin right after a meal. With each additional dose, the intensity of the flush begins to decrease. With time, most people stop being bothered by the flush, even as they gradually increase their niacin intake.

I have found that the best way for me to accurately control the flushing sensation is to start with very small amounts of niacin and gradually increase until the first flush is noticed. One method is to start with a mere 25 mg three times a day, say with each meal. The next day, try 50 mg at breakfast, 25 mg at lunch, and 25 mg at supper. The following day, try 50 mg at breakfast, 50 mg at lunch, and 25 mg at supper. And, the next day, 50 mg at each of the three meals. The next day, 75, 50, and 50, and so on. Continue to increase the dosage by 25 mg per day until the flush occurs.

It is difficult to predict an initial saturation level for niacin, because each person is different. Experience will show you better than I can tell you.

Now that you've had your first flush, what next? Since a flush indicates saturation of niacin, it is desirable to continue to repeat the flushing, just very slightly, to continue the saturation. This could be done three or more times per day.

Safety of High-Dose Niacin

An important point here is that niacin is a vitamin, not a drug. It is not habit forming. Niacin does not require a prescription because it is that safe. It is a nutrient that everyone needs each day. In his Carl Pfeiffer Memorial Lecture in April 2003, Abram Hoffer, M.D., said, "A person's upper limit is that amount which causes nausea, and, if not reduced, vomiting. The dose should never be allowed to remain at its upper limit. The usual therapeutic range is 3,000 to 9,000 milligrams daily in divided doses, but occasionally some patients may need more. The toxic dose for dogs is about 6,000 milligrams per kilogram of body weight. That is equivalent to over a half pound of niacin per day for a human. No human takes 225,000 milligrams of niacin a day. They would be nauseous long before reaching a harmful dose. We do not know the toxic dose for humans since niacin has never killed anyone. The top niacin dose ever was a sixteen-year-old schizophrenic girl who took 120 tablets (500 mg each) in one day. That is 60,000 mg of niacin. The 'voices' she had been hearing were gone immediately. She then took 3,000 mg a day to maintain wellness. Niacin is probably not quite as safe as water, but pretty close to it."

Safe, and very effective. The most mentally disturbed person I've personally worked with was a suicidal lady who spent her life sitting facing the corner, refusing to talk to anyone. On 12,000 mg of niacin daily, she was sitting at the dinner table, happily chatting with her family.

Inevitable physician skepticism and questions about niacin's proven safety and effectiveness are best answered in Dr. Hoffer's books and in *Orthomolecular Psychiatry,* edited by David Hawkins and Linus Pauling. This 700-page textbook is the standard reference for details on megavitamin therapy. People with a history of heavy alcohol use, liver disorders, diabetes, or pregnancy will especially want to have their physician monitor their use of niacin in quantity. Monitoring long-term use of niacin is a good idea for anyone. It consists of having your doctor check your liver function with a simple blood test. It also involves correct interpretation of liver function tests. "Niacin is not liver toxic," says Dr. Hoffer. "Niacin therapy increases liver function tests. But this elevation means that the liver is active. It does not indicate an underlying liver pathology." Dr. Hoffer's voice needs to be heeded. He has treated 5,000 patients with high-dose niacin over a period of fifty years.

Helpful Hints

Niacin may be purchased in tablets at any pharmacy or health-food store. Tablets typically are available in 50 mg, 100 mg, or 250 mg doses. The tablets are usually scored down the middle so you can break them in half easily.

If niacin is taken right after a meal, the flush may be delayed. In fact, the flush may occur long enough afterwards that you forget about it! Don't let the flush surprise you. Remember that niacin does that, and you can control it easily. If you want a flush right away, you can powder the niacin tablet. This is easily done by crushing it between two spoons. Powdered niacin on an empty stomach can result in a flush within minutes.

Other Forms of Niacin

Sustained-release niacin is often advertised as not causing a flush at all. This is not completely true; sometimes the flush is just postponed. It would probably be difficult to determine your saturation level with a product like this. It is also more costly.

Inositol hexaniacinate is a form of "flush-free" niacin. It is more expensive than regular niacin, but is ideal for people who simply cannot abide flushing. It is also called "inositol hexanicotinate." You should know that "nicotinate" is strictly a chemical name; niacin has nothing biologically to do with nicotine.

Niacinamide is the form of niacin found in multivitamins and B-complex preparations. Niacinamide does not cause a flush at all, even at the very highest doses. However, high doses of niacinamide tend to cause nausea sooner than do high doses of regular niacin. In my opinion, it is less effective in inducing relaxation. Also, niacinamide does not lower serum cholesterol. Inositol hexaniacinate does. This is an important distinction to make when purchasing.

The B Complex

It is a good idea to take all the other B-complex vitamins in a separate supplement in addition to the niacin. The B vitamins, like basketball players, work best as a team. Still, the body seems to need proportionally more niacin than the other B vitamins. Even the RDA for niacin is much more than for any other B vitamin. Many physicians consider the current RDA for niacin of only 20 mg to be way too low for optimum health. While the government continues to discuss this, it is possible to decide for yourself, based on the success of doctors that use niacin for their patients every day.

Recommended Reading

Hawkins DR and Pauling L. *Orthomolecular Psychiatry.* San Francisco: Freeman, 1973.

Hoffer A. *Vitamin B₃ and Schizophrenia: Discovery, Recovery, Controversy.* Kingston, ON: Quarry Press, 1998.

Vitamin C Megadose Therapy

Vitamin C has varying activity in the body at varying levels of intake. At low levels of consumption, vitamin C is like a trace nutrient: you need very little of it to stay alive, but without any at all you die. Even a few mg a day will suffice to preserve life. At moderate levels of consumption—say 500–1,500 mg per day for an adult—the vitamin works to build health. Fewer colds will be reported; incidence, severity, and duration of influenza will be less. But it is at high levels—8,000–40,000 mg per day—that we begin to obtain therapeutic properties for the vitamin.

At this high level, vitamin C has antihistamine, antitoxin, antiviral, and antibiotic properties. The pharmacological effects of a vitamin at high concentration do not disqualify our continuing to call it, and think of it, as a vitamin. Money still buys things even if you have a lot of it; its nature has not changed, but its power has. If it takes 100 gallons of gas to drive from New York City to Los Angeles, you simply are not going to make it on 10 gallons, no matter how you try. Likewise, if your body wants 70,000 mg of vitamin C to fight an infection, 7,000 mg won't do. The key is to take enough C, take it often enough, and take it long enough.

The safety of vitamin C is extraordinary, even in enormously high doses. Compared to commonly used prescription drugs, side effects are virtually nonexistent. I do not know of a single case of vitamin C toxicity anywhere in the world's medical literature. The major side effect of vitamin C overload is an unmistakable, urgent diarrhea. This indicates absolute saturation, and the daily dose is then promptly dropped to the highest amount that will not bring about diarrhea. That is a *therapeutic* level. Robert Cathcart, M.D., routinely employs high–ascorbic acid therapy with his patients with success. Frederick Klenner, M.D., has seen cures of diphtheria, staph and strep infections, herpes, mumps, spinal meningitis, mononucleosis, shock, viral hepatitis, arthritis, and polio using high doses of vitamin C. Dr. Klenner says, "Ascorbic acid is the safest and the most valuable substance available to the physician."

How much vitamin C is an effective therapeutic dose? Bowel tolerance. Physicians have administered as much as 200,000 mg per day. Generally, a therapeutic dose will be in the neighborhood of 350–700 mg per kilogram body weight per day. That is a lot of vitamin C. But then again, the goal is success, not political correctness. Physicians experienced with vitamin C all emphasize that small amounts do not work.

Perhaps the biggest misconception about vitamin C therapy is the assumption that one size fits all. It most certainly doesn't. Sicker bodies hold vastly more vitamin C than do healthy bodies.

Some people need to buffer their vitamin C if they have a sensitive tummy. You can take your C with a calcium-magnesium supplement, or with a little bicarbonate of soda, or use an already-buffered form of vitamin C such as calcium ascorbate.

The safety and effectiveness of high vitamin C doses have been well established by medical physicians and decades of practice. Before accepting scare stories about ascorbic acid, you should investigate for yourself. If you haven't yet read the books listed below, you don't know what you're missing. Additionally, you and your doctor may well wish to read papers by William McCormick, M.D., Linus Pauling, Ph.D., Abram Hoffer, M.D., and Robert Cathcart III, M.D. *The Journal of Orthomolecular Medicine* is especially recommended.

How to Get to a Therapeutic Level of Vitamin C

As I always say, "Take enough C to be symptom-free, whatever the amount might be." It's corny, but it works. The effective therapeutic level is also known as "saturation" or "bowel tolerance." Gradually increase your daily vitamin C dose until you have, or are on the verge of having, diarrhea. Vitamin C diarrhea is frequent, watery, and explosive. You may find that you do not have to get quite to that point to reach saturation. Try this: when you feel (or hear) a rumbling or gurgling in the bowel, back off the amount of C that got you there. You are now probably close to bowel tolerance.

Again you ask, why so much? Simply put, this is the quantity that gets results. At saturation levels, vitamin C has strong antibiotic, antihistamine, antiviral, and antipyretic effects. That means that a saturation level kills bacteria, reduces congestion, inactivates viruses, and lowers fevers.

It cannot be overemphasized that very large quantities of vitamin C are required if you want it to work against real illnesses. You don't take the amount of vitamin C you *think* you should need; you take the amount that does the job!

If you are taking large doses of vitamin C, and decide for any reason to stop doing so, I think it is important to *gradually* decrease the daily dose. This is best done over a week or two. An abrupt halt leaves the body in a lurch. A pilot gradually reduces the airspeed of a jet as the runway approaches; abrupt landings are not appreciated by the passengers. Avoiding sudden drops in your vitamin C level prevents a rebound effect where temporary vitamin C deficiency symptoms occur.

"Do I have to stay at saturation forever?" is another common question. The answer is, yes, yes, and no. Yes, in that you need to stay at or just below bowel tolerance as long as you are ill. The second "yes" is that bowel tolerance is self-adjusting. As a person gets better, he gets to saturation sooner and the dose comes down. A sick body holds an enormous amount of vitamin C. A healthy body holds much less. So the 70,000 mg of C that barely caused a fart when you had influenza would be a toilet-shattering catastrophe when you are in good health. So the real answer is, in effect, "no." As you get better, your saturation dose automatically decreases.

Isn't this neat? And you can monitor the entire process on your own.

Objections to Vitamin C Megadoses

Many people wonder, in the face of strong evidence for vitamin C's efficacy, why the medical profession has not embraced vitamin C therapy with open and grateful arms. The reason is this: many studies that claim to "test" vitamin effectiveness are designed to disprove it.

You can set up any experiment to fail. One way to ensure failure is to make a meaningless test. A meaningless test is assured if you make the choice to use inappropriate administration of insufficient quantities of the substance to be investigated.

If I were to give every homeless person I met on the street 25 cents, I could easily prove that money will not help poverty. If a nutrition study uses less than 20,000 or 30,000 mg of vitamin C, it is unlikely to show any antihistamine, antibiotic, or antiviral benefit whatsoever. You have to give enough to get the job done. As long as such research as is done uses piddling little doses of vitamins, doses that are invariably too small to work, megavitamin therapy will be touted as "unproven."

Probably the main roadblock to studies of megavitamin therapy is the widespread belief that there must be unknown dangers to tens of thousands of milligrams of ascorbic acid. Yet, since the time such therapy was introduced in the 1940s by Frederick Klenner, M.D., and up to the present, there has been a surprisingly safe and effective track record to follow. One death from vitamin overdose occurs about every ten years in the United States. According to Lucian Leape, in a 1994 *JAMA* article, "Error in Medicine," there are more than 100,000 pharmaceutical drug deaths annually in America. By this yardstick, vitamins are literally one million times safer than medicines.

On top of this, several reported side effects of vitamin C have been found to be completely mythical. According to a NIH report published in *JAMA* in April 1999, *none* of the following problems are caused by taking too much vitamin C: Hypoglycemia, rebound scurvy, infertility, and destruction of vitamin B_{12}.

Safety and effectiveness should always be the benchmark for any therapeutic program. When one considers that even the AMA admits to more than 100,000 deaths annually from routine administration of prescription drugs, I think we need to consider anew the merits of truly large doses of vitamin C.

Bioflavonoids and Vitamin C

So what exactly is a rose hip, anyway? Any biologist knows that roses don't have hips because they are not vertebrates. Ha! Actually, rose hips are the fruit of a rose bush. All flowers give rise to fruits, and the rose is no exception. When I hike, I look for wild or feral rosebushes and munch on the hips as soon as they are ready (usually early autumn). They are often found on the bushes throughout the entire winter, just waiting for you to come along. Eaten fresh or dried, they are good sources of vitamin C.

Rose hips are also a rich source of bioflavonoids, plant compounds that improve uptake and utilization of vitamin C. Albert Szent-Györgyi won the Nobel prize for his research with vitamin C and related factors back in the 1930s. He actually proposed the term "vitamin P" for the "protective" phytochemicals in bioflavonoids. In a rather adorable, unplanned bit of research, Szent-Györgyi was feeding pure vitamin C to his lab mice when one evening some of them snuck out of their cage and ate his dinner when he wasn't looking. The meal consisted of stuffed green peppers. Szent-Györgyi observed that the animals that ate the peppers seemed to require considerably less ascorbic acid than the other critters. Peppers, along with many fruits and vegetables, are high in bioflavonoids.

This bioflavonoid–vitamin C connection is why you often see "rose hip" vitamin C tablets offered for sale. Here is the kicker, though: there is so very little rose hips powder in most such tablets that it is a waste of money to pay extra for what amounts to zilch. I (in agreement with Linus Pauling) recommend that people buy the cheapest vitamin C they can find, and take a lot of it. In addition, people need to eat right—lots of fruits and veggies. Fruits and veggies are a mediocre source of vitamin C but an excellent source of bioflavonoids. Vitamin C tablets are a lousy source of bioflavonoids, but a good source of C. Good match.

Recommended Reading

Townsend Letter for Doctors, April, 1992.

Drug Abuse Warning Network (DAWN) Statistical Series I, Number 9, Annual Data 1989.

Leape L. Error in medicine. *Journal of the American Medical Association,* 272 (1994): 1851.

Levy T. *Vitamin C, Infectious Diseases, and Toxins: Curing the Incurable.* Philadelphia, PA: Xlibris, 2002.

Hughes RE and Jones PR. Natural and synthetic sources of vitamin C. *J Sci Food Agric* 22 (1971): 551–52.

Jones E and Hughes RE. The influence of bioflavonoids on the absorption of vitamin C. *IRCS Med Sci* 12 (1984): 320.

Vinson JA and Bose P. Comparative bioavailability of synthetic and natural vitamin C in Guinea pigs. *Nutr Rep Intl* 27 (1983): 875.

Vinson JA and Bose P. Comparative bioavailability to humans of ascorbic acid alone or in a citrus extract. *Am J Clin Nutr* 48 (1988): 6014.

Cathcart RF, III The method of determining proper doses of vitamin C for the treatment of disease by titrating to bowel tolerance. *Journal of Orthomolecular Psychiatry* 10 (1981a): 125–32.

Cheraskin E, et al. *The Vitamin C Connection.* New York: Harper and Row, 1983.

McCormick WJ. Lithogenesis and hypovitaminosis. *Medical Record* 159 (1946): 410–13.

Pauling L. *How to Live Longer and Feel Better.* San Francisco: W. H. Freeman, 1986.

Pauling L. *Vitamin C, the Common Cold, and the Flu.* San Francisco: W. H. Freeman, 1976.

Smith LH, ed. *Clinical Guide to the Use of Vitamin C.* [This is a summary of Dr. Frederick Klenner's published papers.] Tacoma, WA: Life Sciences Press, 1988.

Stone I. *The Healing Factor: Vitamin C Against Disease.* New York: Putnam, 1972.

How to Get Intravenous Vitamin C Given to a Hospitalized Patient

For very serious illnesses, parenteral (infused or injected) administration of vitamin C is more effective than even the largest of oral doses. While I personally have seen aggressive oral doses beat illnesses as bad as viral pneumonia, the vitamin C specialists (such as William McCormick, Frederick Klenner, Robert Cathcart, and Hugh Riordan) all give megavitamin C therapy by intravenous infusion or intramuscular injection. Since electing this procedure necessarily makes you dependent on a doctor, I have some very specific ideas and instructions as to how you can arrange for an IV of vitamin C.

1. **Know before you go.** It is immeasurably easier to get what you want if you contract for it beforehand. Prenuptial agreements, new car deals, roofing and siding estimates, and hospital care need to be negotiated in advance. When the tow truck comes, it is too late to complain about who's driving. Same with an ambulance, or a hasty hospital admission. You have to pre-plan, and here's how:

2. **Get a letter.** Yes, a "note from the doctor" still carries clout. Have your general practitioner sign a letter stating that he backs your request for a vitamin C IV drip, 10 grams per 12 hours, should you (or your designated loved one) require hospitalization. Have copies made and keep them handy. Update the letter annually. You now have your G.P.'s permission. Good start, but not enough.

3. **Get some more letters.** Try to obtain a similar letter from every specialist that you have used, are using, or may use in the foreseeable future. This sounds cumbersome, but is no more unmanageable than most people's grocery lists. Keep it in perspective: this is just as important as wearing a medical-alert bracelet or keeping a fresh battery in Grandpa's pacemaker.

4. **Make some calls.** Telephone a representative or two from every hospital within fifty miles of your home. Find out which wants your business the most. When you find a "live one" on the phone, write down their name and title, and follow up with a letter.

5. **Write for your rights.** In your letter, ask for the hospital's permission to have a vitamin C IV drip, infusion, push, or injection, as well as oral vitamin C, should you or

your designated family member(s) come in to that hospital. *You must get this in writing.* Now, do *not* say, "I want that in writing," because people do not like that. But if you write to them by U.S. Mail, they will naturally write back to you. Bingo. Don't correspond by e-mail; you want a real signature on hospital letterhead.

You might be wondering, What if they write back, "No, we won't." Hold onto that letter. You can make a real stink with it should you need to play hardball in court, and I don't mean a handball court. More likely, however, they simply won't write back. Would you entrust your life to a hospital that refuses to even answer their mail? Make a point to go somewhere else. If you live in a rural community or smaller city, you might be thinking that you do not have a choice of hospitals. But people can be moved. It happens all the time.

What is most likely is that the hospital's representative will send you a garbage answer, so noncommittal as to be unusable. Try this: have your doctor "write" the letter. The doctor's letterhead and signature; your composition. You can give a professional a rough draft of what you want said. I had a lawyer ask me to do exactly that when I sought (and succeeded in getting) a vitamin C IV for my hospitalized father. I wrote it and faxed it to the attorney; his staff rewrote it on his stationery and he signed it. It saves time. Be sure your doctor's letter clearly requests a reply.

It is also quite possible that they will ask for more information. This could be a genuine interest, but it is more likely a stall. If you think Nero fiddled while Rome burned, you should see what medical bureaucrats can do. To cut through the treacle, you need to understand the nature of the beast. The first rule of lion taming is, You have to know more than the lions. Therefore:

6. **Know the law.** Many states have enacted legislation that makes it possible for a physician to provide any natural therapy that a patient requests without fear of losing his or her license. If your state has such a law, it will make it easier to get a doctor to prescribe a vitamin C IV.

7. **Know the power structure.** Find out who is in charge. I have heard doctors say that they'd be happy to start a vitamin C IV, but the hospital will not let them. Then, when asked, I have heard the hospital say that they allow vitamin C IVs but the doctors won't do them. To avoid an endless Catch-22 situation, you have to know the ropes and where everybody stands. Go to the person that can do you the most good (or harm) and start your negotiations there. If you can persuade the king, the castle is yours.

On the hospital side, which of the administrators has the clout? Talk to their secretaries (they are the people who really run things anyway) and you will find out. It could be that the most influential person for you may be the hospital's patient rights advocate or VP for customer service. It might even be the public relations director. Who knows? You sure don't, so remove the veil of anonymity and find out.

The patient, if conscious, has all the power because it is her body. If a patient

195

insists loud and long enough, she can get almost anything. Since patients tend to be sick, and therefore easily slip into becoming noncombatants, a family member has to get in there and pitch for them. A highly experienced nurse told me that she would never leave a family member in a hospital without a twenty-four-hour-a-day guard in the form of a friend or family member or other advocate. That is sound advice from a lady who's seen it.

Next to the patient, the most powerful family member is the spouse. After that, it would be children. You do not have to have power of attorney, but it helps. If the patient is unable to speak, act, or think, it may be essential. Do not wait until the patient is incapacitated to plan this. Your family needs to come together and present a preplanned, unified front to the medical and administrative people. You may think I am overstating the case, but I have seen patients die simply because no one took the reins and got the C in the veins. I have seen vitamin C IVs halted simply because the patient was moved to intensive care. Think that one over. I have seen vitamin C prescriptions overruled by a nurse or pharmacist. You would not think that possible, would you? Well, it is. There is no nice way to phrase this. Stay on top of the situation or you will have a premature burial on your hands.

8. **Know your recourse.** If you are rich, get your lawyer on the phone. Better yet, bring your lawyer to the hospital. If you are like the rest of us, you may simply have to bluff if you threaten to call your attorney. The purpose here is to save the life of your loved one, not to make a buck from a malpractice suit. Personally, I think malpractice suits are a sign of the most abject failure on the part of the family, as well as the medical profession. In the same way that accident insurance does not prevent accidents but only pays the costs, so do malpractice settlements fail to resuscitate a dead family member. "Death control" is somewhat like birth control in that you have to act before the event takes place.

9. **Know the facts about vitamin C IVs.** For this, there is absolutely no alternative to reading up on the subject. You will want to begin with medical papers written by Frederick Klenner, Robert Cathcart, Ewan Cameron, and Hugh Riordan. This book's bibliography contains many titles you can begin with.

10. **Know how to avoid the run-around.** Doctors and hospitals are quick to offer rather bogus reasons why they would deny your request for a vitamin C IV. Each of these arguments is a lot of bull, and easily refuted.

    Their argument: "We do not have Vitamin C for intravenous infusion in our pharmacy."

    Your response: "So get some. Or just make it yourselves." (Instructions on how to prepare it, written by a highly experienced physician, can be found at DoctorYourself.com.)

196

Their argument: "We've never done this before."

Your response: "Then this is a wonderful opportunity to learn. I've never lost a (insert family member's position here) before."

Their argument: "The patient is too ill."

Your response: "That's why we want the vitamin C IV."

Their argument: "We might get into trouble if we do this."

Your response: "You will be in legal trouble for sure if you don't."

Their argument: "There is no scientific evidence that this is safe, effective, appropriate for this case, blah, blah, blah . . ."

Your response: "Read this." (This short phrase is to be spoken as you produce a large stack of actual studies written by medical doctors who have successfully used vitamin C IVs. See references mentioned above.)

Their argument: "But we do not have time to read all those papers."

Your response: "That's okay. I already have, and it's my body (or my father's, or my mother's). Run the vitamin C IV. Start with 10 grams every 12 hours and do not stop it without my written authorization."

Their argument: "This hospital operates under our authority, these are our rules, and this is the way it is done."

Your response: "This is my mother. If you deny her the treatment the family requests, you will be sued, and we will win. Do you really want to go to the wall on this one?"

Confrontational? Yes. But I have seen too many people die too soon. Frederick Klenner was right when he said, "Some physicians would stand by and see their patient die rather than use ascorbic acid."

Don't let it happen to your family.

Juicing

Infomercials do nothing for me personally, but the ones for juicers are in the main correct: juicing makes you healthier and makes you feel better. The first is a long-term observation, the second you can see for yourself in a few days.

Why not just eat all those vegetables raw? Because you won't, that's why. I often juice five pounds or more of carrots, plus six to eight apples, just for breakfast. I'd never find the time to eat all that without the shortcut of a juicer. Also, your body's absorption of fresh, raw juice is simply outstanding. A juicer is essentially a powerful motor with teeth. It breaks cell walls and releases all the plant's nutrients into a solution that your body sucks up like a sponge. Having taught cell biology for so long, I've become familiar with what that good stuff is: plant RNA and DNA (no, this will not grow leaves on your nose), cytoplasm, mitochondria, ribosomes, enzymes and coenzymes, vitamins and minerals, plus the usual proteins, lipids, and carbohydrates. Juicing gives you the lot, and all uncooked, which is important since cooking destroys many beneficial enzymes in raw foods.

I've been juicing for decades now, and have seen it change many lives besides my own. I have also heard two frequent complaints:

1. *"The juicer and the vegetables cost too much!"* Simple answer: A brake job on your car is three hundred dollars. That will get you a really good juicer—which will serve just as important a role in protecting your health. But if you just have to get that brake job first, you can go cheap to start with. I've picked up cheap juicers, new, for as little as $20. Garage sales are a resource for used ones. (Concerned about sanitation? Common household bleach will clean and disinfect plastic and metal juicer parts to a surgical nurse's satisfaction.) The cost of the produce is no more than you'd spend on other foods that aren't even good for you. I've seen people at the supermarket check out two ritzy cuts of meat and not blink an eye at the $50 it cost them. You couldn't even fit fifty bucks of carrots in a grocery cart. Garden, and the price plummets further.

2. *"Juicing takes too much time!"* Simple answer: No, it doesn't. It takes no more time than fixing a regular meal, and probably less. How much time do you spend in doc-

tors' waiting rooms? In line at the checkout? Watching TV? C'mon, everybody has a little time for their health.

The carotene in one cup of carrot juice is probably the equivalent of nearly 20,000 IU of vitamin A. So there's one nutrient you surely do not need to buy as a supplement. It's also worth noting that carotene in high doses has been shown to strengthen the immune system by helping the body to build more helper T cells.

Excess carotene causes the skin to turn slightly orange, once succinctly described in a newspaper as resembling an artificial suntan. This is harmless. Vitamin-A toxicity is possible from the preformed, oil type of vitamin A, but not from carotene. In short, it is singularly difficult to kill yourself with carrots. Or juice.

Hints

I'm no Heloise, but by this point I've become a middling–fair juicing expert. Here are some tips for making your juicing experience a rewarding one.

To get more juice, reduce clogging, and simplify cleanup, add some peeled zucchini along with your carrots. My "Carrottini" (trademark!) juice tastes better than it sounds.

If there is a "head" of frothy foam on the top of your glass of juice, you can either enjoy the taste and milkshake-like texture of it (I do), or avoid it by drinking through a straw.

If the leftover vegetable pulp produced by your juicer seems damp or wet, you may be pushing vegetables through too fast. Take your time and let the machine do its job. Use only a subtle pressure, with the plunger supplied by the manufacturer, to send the produce through your juicer. Taking your time juicing can yield as much as a third more juice. It will also reduce the heat from pressing vegetables too hard against the juicer's blade assembly. Reduced friction means cooler juice, which is to be preferred. To this end, I frost up a couple of large drinking glasses, and the glass pitcher I collect the juice in, by sticking them in the freezer each night. Next morning, I begin. Naturally, refrigerating (but NOT freezing!) your fresh produce also keeps everything cooler.

Twice a year, juice a couple of pounds of grapes with seeds to clean the innards of the juicer. I like to use concord grapes, and afterwards let the juice sit for, oh, about five days. And *then* I drink it. Oh yeah!

Add a tablespoon or two of frozen natural juice concentrates (especially lemonade, grape, or pineapple) to kill the taste of any juice you do not like. Try it with cucumber or cabbage. Another way is to have a chaser ready. Pick your very favorite, sweet juice and have a full glass ready as your reward for first drinking the good-for-you vegetable juice.

If your family runs for cover at first sight of your intent to liquefy everything in the fridge, then snag your dog. Our dog's ears perk up at the sound of a Champion revving up, for she knows that the vegetable pulp is all for her. We mix it with her dog food to greatly increase its vegetable, vitamin, and fiber content. It is also low-calorie and filling, so it keeps her thin. No dog? Then put the pulp in your compost pile. No compost pile? Well, why not? Okay, okay, one more option: carrot pulp is just the ticket for carrot cake. And that might even get your family back into the kitchen again.

Clean the clogs as you go. Carrots and other veggies can be very fibrous at certain times of the year. If you are really going at it, stop juicing every five pounds or so, unplug the juicer, and (carefully) rinse the blade assembly under running cold tap water. No soap needed.

Recommended Reading

Alexander M, et al. Oral beta-carotene can increase the number of OKT4 cells in human blood. *Immunology Letters* 9 (1985): 221–24.

Tang AM, et al. Dietary micronutrient intake and risk of progression to acquired immunodeficiency syndrome (AIDS) in human immunodeficiency virus type 1 (HIV-1)-infected homosexual men. *Am J Epidemiol* 138 (1993): 937–51.

Breakfast Blast

I like to start the day with a quart and a half of carrot juice. It is carrot-and-zucchini in summer and carrot-and-apple in autumn. Off season, however, I am more likely to get my start with a breakfast concoction I lovingly call "slurry." Here's the recipe:

Breakfast "Slurry"

One pint fruit juice
*(Orange juice from frozen concentrate works fine
and is frequently on sale. Pineapple juice is great, too.
Buy unsweetened, bearing in mind that it is naturally,
intensely sweet. And that's just as well, given
what you're going to put into it.)*

Three (or more) rounded tablespoons lecithin granules

One teaspoon vitamin C crystals
(approximately 4,500 mg)

Mix together in a spacious stein, and chug-a-lug!

I also take the following supplements everyday, whether it's with the veggie juice or with the "slurry." If you're an average-weight male, you can do the same. Others can modify this to match their weight.

- 600 IU vitamin E (as natural mixed tocopherols, containing 80 percent d-alpha-tocopherol)

- 100–200 mg niacin (more if I don't flush, less if I do)

- 3 calcium-magnesium tablets (each supplying about 200 mg calcium and 100 mg magnesium. This also helps buffer the vitamin C)

- 5 multiple digestive enzyme tablets (to help your tummy more easily handle the lecithin. Pancreatin will do, although it is not vegetarian. Vegetarian enzyme sources, which usually include papaya and other fruits, cost more.)

- 1 high-potency multivitamin, providing:

- 400 IU vitamin D

- 25 mg thiamine (vitamin B_1)

- 25 mg riboflavin (vitamin B_2)

- 100 mg niacinamide (vitamin B_3)

- 25 mg pyridoxine (vitamin B_6)

- 400 mcg folic acid

- 25 mcg vitamin B_{12}

- 200 mcg biotin

- 25 mg pantothenic acid

- 15 mg zinc

- 25 mcg selenium

- 4 mg manganese

- 25 mcg chromium

(The multivitamin also contains moderate additional amounts of vitamins A, C, and E. If the multivitamin's mineral quantities seem on the low side, bear in mind that I take this multivitamin again at lunch, and again at dinner, for total of three a day. I also take an additional 60 mg of zinc and 200 mcg of chromium at lunchtime.)

After I scarf all this down, I enjoy a chaser cup of undoctored fruit juice. I am now good for six hours or more without any food or any hunger.

I must express a debt of gratitude to Dr. Jacobus Rinse, whose famous Rinse Formula is the basis for my modification presented above.

202

Vitamin B$_{12}$ Supplementation

L et's set the matter straight from the start: If you do not like getting shots of B$_{12}$, you should be aware that intranasal absorption (discussed below) is the next best thing. Oral administration of B$_{12}$ supplements is largely ineffective. This goes for so-called sublingual B$_{12}$ tablets as well.

Vitamin B$_{12}$, unlike other B vitamins, is stored in muscle and other organs of the body. A little B$_{12}$ goes a long way, what is stored lasts a long time, and it may take years to deplete your body's reserves. But sooner or later, usually later (after age forty), not only do poor eating habits catch up with us, but we also lose the ability to efficiently absorb what B$_{12}$ we do get from food.

Cobalamin is the proper name for vitamin B$_{12}$. It is a really huge molecule (C$_{63}$H$_{90}$O$_{14}$PCo). The "Co" is for the one cobalt atom at its core. B$_{12}$ is obtained mostly, but not exclusively, by eating animal products such as dairy and meat. Grass-and-grain-eating cattle get their B$_{12}$ from synthesis by microorganisms in their gastrointestinal tract. Yes, B$_{12}$ is also synthesized in the human GI tract, but not enough. It can be enhanced by a good vegetarian diet that favors an internal population of beneficial, B$_{12}$-making bacteria, but we still need more than that. Nutritional yeast, fermented soy foods such as tempeh, and sprouts (according to some sources) are vegetarian sources of dietary B$_{12}$.

Absorption of dietary B$_{12}$ takes place in the very last part of the small intestine, right before the colon. Absorption requires a biochemical helper molecule called "intrinsic factor," which is a glycoprotein normally secreted by cells lining your stomach. Strong stomach hydrochloric acid is also required to split up this huge molecule. (That's why a weak acid like vitamin C (ascorbic acid) is harmless to B$_{12}$, persistent myths to the contrary). Even sublingual (under-the-tongue) B$_{12}$ supplements are probably ineffective because the cobalamin molecule is too large to diffuse through the mucosa of the mouth. And if your body no longer makes intrinsic factor like it should, you cannot absorb oral B$_{12}$ supplements very well, either.

The end result can be pernicious anemia, which is more than the classic inability to make enough hemoglobin for your red blood cells. Pernicious anemia also results in a sore mouth and tongue, assorted burning and tingling sensations, and eventually neurological damage. I think Ménière's syndrome and dementia symptoms mistaken for Alzheimer's disease might be a manifestation of this as well.

While there is a urine test for B_{12} deficiency, to get accurate B_{12} readings it is necessary to measure the cerebrospinal fluid. If you are not a spinal tap fan, consider a simple, noninvasive therapeutic trial of B_{12}. This is so inexpensive and safe that it would be difficult to deny it to anyone. I would suggest your doctor try a 1,000 mcg injection at least once a week. Compared to the RDA of only about 3 mcg, that dose may appear hefty. But given the miserable nature of unappreciated B_{12} deficiency diseases, erring on the high side may be preferable to unnecessarily delaying recovery. And I know of no side effects whatsoever with B_{12} overdose.

Intranasal (that is, by way of the nose) administration sounds pretty weird, but it is an efficient delivery method for large-sized molecules whether you like the sound of it or not. Your nose has two choices:

1. Buy ready-to-use, over-the-counter B_{12} gel, which you will occasionally find for sale in a pharmacy or health-food store. Some products come in individual disposable packets. These are pricey.

2. Make your own B_{12} intranasal supplement. It is cheap, easy, and best done behind closed doors. Obtain your doctor's okay before trying this procedure. Take any B_{12} tablet (between 100 to 1,000 mcg) and grind it into a powder between two tablespoons. Add water, just a few drops at a time, to make a soft paste. With a "Q-Tip," it's generic equivalent, or your clean pinkie finger, gently swab the paste inside your nose up to a comfortable level. Do not push; use no force whatsoever. The excipients (tableting ingredients) are more likely to bother your schnoz than the B_{12} is. If it irritates you, try using less, or a different brand of tablet. I'd try this two times a week for a month.

Feel free to quit at any time and get B_{12} shots instead. Once in a great while doctors will even teach you how to give yourself B_{12} shots, but that remains a singularly rare event. Hence this nose news.

Stress Reduction

Frequently in this book I've suggested stress reduction as one key to alleviating many health problems. You already know some things you should be doing, or not doing, in order to relieve stress. Here is my three-step plan for even better results.

Step One: Experience Relaxation

It does no good to tell somebody to relax. They need to be shown how to relax, immediately and reliably. For me, the end of tension began with a book. That particular book was *Relief without Drugs,* by Australian psychiatrist Ainslie Meares. Shortly thereafter, I began to do a technique known as progressive relaxation. It is time-honored, easy, and works surprisingly well. Here's the version I learned in the psychiatric wing of Canberra Hospital as a visiting student:

While sitting with your eyes closed, pay attention to your toes. Yes, *those* toes. Relax your toes. Really relax them, too. If you do not know what this means, tense them up and *then* relax them. Then, without tensing, relax them some more. Next, relax the soles of your feet in the same way. Then your ankles. Then your calves. Then thighs, hips, abdomen, and so forth. Relax each region of your body as you progress upward, ending with your head. Relaxing each part of the face is especially effective. Keeping your eyes closed, feel how relaxed you are. Feel your whole body relaxed. Feel your mind relaxed. Now just sit and enjoy it for a few minutes. Then slowly open your eyes, take a deep breath or two, and off you go.

Step Two: Regular Practice Brings Progress

State University of New York emeritus professor of biology John Mosher has provided the following six suggestions for a breath-based method of stress reduction, which you may find even more profoundly settling than Step One was. Because this practice is very settling and relaxing, it is best done before eating, in the morning and evening.

1. Choose a quiet comfortable place. It is best to do the meditation sitting up with your back comfortably straight.

2. With eyes closed, be aware of your breathing. Be sure you are breathing from the

diaphragm ("belly breathing") and not the chest. Your lower abdominal area should easily rise and fall as you inhale and exhale.

3. Try some "alternating breathing." The alternating breathing simply consists of breathing through one nostril at a time. Use your thumb to gently close your right nostril, and inhale through the left nostril. Then, release the right, close the left nostril with your fingers, and now exhale through the right nostril. Then, in through the right nostril, close the right with your thumb, and exhale through the left. Now in with the left, close, and out through the right. Continue this alternating breathing for about five minutes, with the eyes closed.

4. Now discontinue the alternating breathing technique and continue to sit quietly with eyes closed, bringing your attention to your normal breath. Continue to breathe from the diaphragm.

5. Be mindful of inhaling and exhaling. Continue this "mindful" breathing for fifteen or twenty minutes. If during the breathing your mind wanders and gets off on thoughts, as soon as you realize your attention is not on the breathing, very gently turn your attention from the thought to the breathing. Do not try to control your thoughts! Do not dwell on thoughts.

6. At the end of fifteen or twenty minutes of the "mindful" breathing, lie down and relax with eyes closed for ten minutes. At the end of your rest, come back into activity very gradually and easily.

Step Three: Centering Prayer

Contemplatives and scholars alike have pointed out that many religious and secular traditions share an interest in stress reduction that may be gained from meditation or prayer. One widely practiced faith-based technique is known as Centering Prayer, or Prayer of the Heart. The following books discuss and describe this method:

Bacovcin H, trans. *The Way of a Pilgrim and the Pilgrim Continues His Way: A New Translation.* New York: Image Books, 1978.

Johnston W, ed. *The Cloud of Unknowing and the Book of Privy Counseling.* New York: Image Books, 1996.

Peers E, trans. Teresa of Avila. *Interior Castle.* New York: Image Books, 1972.

Pennington M. *Daily We Touch Him: Practical Religious Experiences.* Chicago: Sheed and Ward, 1997.

Recommended Reading

Therapeutic meditation is an especially well-researched area of medicine. A free PubMed search (www.nlm.nih.gov) for "meditation" will yield nearly 900 scientific papers on the subject. (And "stress reduction" will get you almost 14,000 matches.)

Scientific Research on the Transcendental Meditation Program: Collected Papers, Volumes 1–6. Fairfield, IA: Maharishi University of Management, 1990.

Evading Exercise

Organized nudity is responsible for it.

When I was a little kid, we boys all swam naked at the YMCA. The one exception was when moms and sisters were invited for special events. I still remember the one kid who forgot it was Family Swim Night and innocently strolled out of the showers and into the pool room in his birthday suit. He did the fastest about-face I've ever seen, and we never let him live it down.

What's more, we were still swimming nude in boy's gym class when I graduated from Charlotte High School in 1970. Back dives were especially revealing. I know this sounds a bit hard to believe, but it was true: nude swimming was the rule all the way through grade twelve in the Rochester, New York public schools. I am reliably informed that the girls got to wear swimsuits in their gym classes.

But not us.

Of course, we all showered together as well. In a scene reminiscent of a juvenile prison movie, after gym class we were compelled to shower. In the scant three minutes given to us for the purpose, enough teen trauma was accumulated to last a lifetime. I mean, how do you cope with such a situation? Everybody had to do it, so evidently we managed. And we learned valuable skills in the process. For example, one of my acquaintances taught me how to get dressed without drying first.

It did not help that my high-school gym teacher took a special dislike to me. I was about 6' 1" and weighed, maybe, 100 pounds. This guy, an obese ex-Marine, was also the wrestling coach. He combined the only two marketable skills he possessed into a brilliant method of selecting sparring teams: he'd line us up by height and have us count off by twos. This meant, of course, that I inevitably ended up with a 6' 1", 220-pound varsity football lineman as my wrestling "partner." I therefore developed the fastest sit-out in wrestling history.

Under such circumstances, it is no surprise that I developed an enduring dislike of all things related to sport. It's not that I haven't tried. Like all the neighborhood boys, I played ball all summer. I mean, that's what boys *did*. My teams never got even remotely close to being in the playoffs, but my brother's did. Which figures.

For the first fifteen years of his life, my older brother was a round-shouldered, horn-rimmed, skinny little twerp. Then he started working out in our basement. Like a mushroom planted in the dark and forgotten, he thrived. Weightlifting utterly transformed him. Good diet, natural maturation, and contact lenses didn't hurt, either, but that Sears and Roebuck weight kit did wonders.

The secret, of course, is that he spent the time using it.

And that brings me to my real point.

You either talk about doing it, or you do it. I do not like to exercise. But I like even less having a pudgy belly, skinny arms, no chest, and health conditions. The health benefits of exercise are vast and well-known. So are the purely physical benefits. That is why I exercise. Of course you and I know it is good to exercise, in the same way that smokers know it is good not to smoke, but knowledge is not enough. You have to do it.

My exercise hints? Thought you'd never ask.

Exercise for a really honest reason: vanity.

Exercise with a friend (or relative, if you are desperate) who has the same goals you do. This is very important for staying on the wagon.

Exercise to music. I recommend the Who, the Rolling Stones, good blues, early Beatles, and maybe a little Badfinger for the rest of you eclectic ex-hippies.

Start small and work up. I began, at my son's insistence, with crunches. When I started, I thought thirty was a lot. After six years, I now do 2,100 crunches in under 50 minutes.

Invest as little money as possible. A cheap exercise bike and a pair of dumbbells is a good start. Maybe add a weight set and a bench. Check garage sales, for a lot of people purchase this stuff, and that act constitutes their entire exercise program: the buying of equipment. Consequently, you can outfit your garage, attic, or basement for very little cash.

But better yet, keep it all in your living room. If you see it, you will use it. Still better, keep all your gear within a remote's distance of your TV. You can watch the tube while you bike. You can kill an hour of brainless network programming and bike miles in the process.

Keep a record. My brother told me that you need to simply beat your own record to be a winner. That's a pretty profound point. I would never have gotten to 2,100 crunches unless I'd wanted to beat 2,000, or 1,000, or 30.

Vary your program. Although I am a crunch-meister, I also use dumbbells for my arms and chest. I happen to already have strong legs from childhood paper routes, chasing my brothers so I'd not be left behind, biking everywhere as a teenager, and living at the top of a hill in Vermont as a car-less young man. So I don't use the bike as much as you might want to. I also walk home with my groceries, and try for a four-mile walk along the nearby Erie Canal on alternate days to my crunching. Again, take a friend, or a dog, for safety, companionship, and mutual encouragement.

Watch the cable exercise channels, especially if you are a beginner. Seeing all those supple, writhing bodies exercising with one great smile is stimulating. Use Richard Simmons exercise tapes, Jane Fonda workout tapes, any workout tapes that appeal to you. Personally, I think the porno industry should come up for air for a minute, and make totally nude workout tapes.

And that brings us full circle: it really *is* all about nudity. Especially how you, with your clothes off, look in the mirror. You will be pleased, your friends will be jealous, and your family will be thrilled to know how much longer they will have you around. Well, they will if you first put your clothes back on.

Weight Loss

Some diets are nothing but quackery.

Sitting through high school chemistry class one gorgeous spring day, an equally bored friend of mine and I came up with a sure-fire diet program based entirely on the thermal properties of water.

Let me run it by you. In eleventh-grade chemistry, we were taught that water has a high specific heat. That is, it takes a lot of heat to raise the temperature of water even a little. A watched pot never boils, or so it seems, because even a gas stove's flames or the red-hot coil of an electric range must work extremely hard to bring that pot up to 212 degrees F. Why? It takes one unit of heat, called a calorie (small "c"), to raise one gram of water (which is one milliliter) by one degree Celsius (1.8 degrees F). Sorry about the math anxiety this may be arousing in you, but I'm going somewhere with this.

Your body temperature is surprisingly hot: 98.6 degrees F, to be exact. "Cold" tap water is perhaps 50 degrees F or less. Ice is 32 degrees F, and "ice water" might be in the high 30s. If ice water were 38.6 degrees, that is fully 60 degrees lower than your body temperature.

Now a dietetic Calorie (with the large C) is more properly termed a kilocalorie, equal to 1,000 small-c calories. It takes 1,000 little one-ml-of-water-one-degree heat calories to make one "food" Calorie.

Hmm. A small-c calorie of heat can only raise one ml of water 1.8 degrees F. A liter of water is 1,000 ml. One food big-C Calorie is 1,000 little calories. So you have to burn one Calorie to raise the temperature of one liter of water 1.8 degrees.

Uh huh. But that means that to raise the temperature of a liter of ice water sixty degrees, to body temperature, takes 33 Calories. Two liters would burn 67 Calories.

We know from dieticians that just 10 extra food Calories per day, for 10 years, will gain you 10 pounds. In other words, if you eat only 10 superfluous Calories each day, you will gain a pound a year. That is admittedly not much. On the other hand, you would have real trouble cutting me a 10-Calorie piece of chocolate cake. On a dessert plate, 10 Calories looks almost insignificant.

If, however, you drink two liters of ice water a day, you will burn 67 Calories each day just heating that water to your normal body temperature. That is almost seven pounds per year weight loss. In ten years, that's 67 pounds of weight lost.

Two liters is just over eight eight-ounce glasses, no more than many a physician would advise you to drink anyway. Make that water cold, and you burn calories watching TV. A pound or so every two months, on ice water. Up it to three liters a day and it's almost a pound a month. No exercise factored in; no dietary changes considered. Just add water. *Cold* water.

But wait, there's more. Many a person drinking more liquids will eat fewer solids. Even water is filling if you drink enough of it. Reduced food means reduced Calories. Take a daily multivitamin tablet to cover the nutrient losses inevitable in any diet. Americans consume more soft drinks than all other beverages put together (yes, that includes milk, tea, coffee, juices, sports drinks, bottled water, liquor, wine, and beer). Drink water instead of pop, and you will be consuming much less sugar (and fewer Calories) or, in the case of diet pop, far less of those questionable artificial sweeteners. You'll also avoid the carbonic acid found in all carbonated beverages, and the phosphoric acid added to colas. Dentists etch teeth with phosphoric acid, and carbonic acid isn't much easier on the enamel.

Can you get too much water? Not easily; your body is naturally mostly water. Your blood is mostly water. Your food is mostly water. Your bowels and kidneys require water for excretion of wastes. Why, you were conceived in an aquatic environment. Too little water is associated with kidney stones, urinary tract infections, febrile illness, dehydration, and worse. So drink yourself slim. Unless your doctor tells you otherwise, two to three liters per day is a reasonable plan.

Just warming up. Vegetable juicing is next.

211

Comedian Dick Gregory came to our college campus to speak against the Vietnam war. The year was 1970, and the controversy was running high. Draft cards were burned and demonstrations shut down classes. I personally saw the student body president, from an overhead stairway, dump the contents of a fifty-pound sack of flour on two Marines at their recruiting table. My hair was a whole lot shorter than the student president's, but a good deal longer than the Marines'. At the time, I was on the student activities lecture committee, and we knew full well we were bringing in a speaker who would be as inflammatory as he was funny. Anything else I knew of Mr. Gregory's politics came from reading *Dick Gregory from the Back of the Bus* a few years earlier.

I was to be surprised. Gregory had pledged not to eat until the war was over. He started his fast at 308 pounds and was down to 135. To save his life, his promise was amended to not eat any solids until the war was over. Vietnam went on for years, so this was no wimp-out. He lived on nothing but juice, fresh vegetable juice. In his lengthy speaking contract were written specifications about which and how many organically grown vegetables we were to provide for him. So our lecture committee went shopping for Mr. Gregory and presented him with two large brown paper bags of fresh food. He carried them right into the Student Union's now very-crowded press conference room, put the overflowing bags on the big walnut table, and casually sat down.

I was four feet away from the man. The room was ablaze with the dazzlingly bright portable white lights of TV reporters. Cameras whirred and clicked and the questions flew. As he quietly answered, Mr. Gregory calmly commenced juicing. I don't quite remember where the juicer came from, but there it was. Cup after cup of orange or green drinks went into the man. The questions from the press stayed on his antiwar views. I don't recall any questions about his diet. It was weird to watch. I thought Mr. Gregory was off his rocker.

Years later, I learned of people weighing 600, 800, even 1,000 pounds losing weight with vegetable juicing when all else had failed. Guess who was behind it? Dick Gregory. He had been called in to get the morbidly obese into vegetable juicing, and did it. He got them doing exactly what he had done, and they lost hundreds of pounds. Plus, they got healthier in the process. Forget his politics; Gregory's enduring contribution will be saved lives.

I myself tried a half-hearted, perhaps one-third vegetable juice diet and lost over twenty pounds in three months. It was easy. Getting someone to try it is the only obstacle.

To summarize: there are four "noble truths" of weight loss.

1. *Fat is real.* And really unhealthy. Half of Americans are overweight, one in four is obese, and over four million are morbidly obese. If you are overweight, admit it now before you die early and miss seeing your grandchildren grow up. Obesity kills 250,000 Americans each year.

2. *Fat has a reason.* If you are overweight, you are either eating too many Calories or burning too few. It's about behaviors, not genetics. If you have heavy parents and you have heavy children, look for what I call dinner table heredity. You are not doomed by your DNA. It is far more likely that you have merely adopted your family's eating habits.

3. *There is a way out.* Behave differently. Eat fewer Calories, or burn more, preferably both. Both are within any human being's power, and don't try to tell me otherwise. Anyone, even a paraplegic, can exercise. Even in a wheelchair or bed you can lift small weights to start. And one of the few genuinely free choices everyone has is what they will or will not put into their mouths.

4. *It's not how much, but what.* Water and vegetable juices are low-calorie and very, very low-fat. There is almost no limit to how much water you can drink, or the amount of vegetables you can eat. Juicing vegetables is even better. Vegetable juicing increases both the quantity of vegetables that you will eat, and increases your absorption of those vegetables. Nutrient deficiency, a common obstacle with dieting, is therefore a nonissue. See my chapters "Saul's Super Remedy" and "Juicing" for more information on juicing.

You cannot live on water alone; Mahatma Gandhi and entirely too many others have approached death after weeks and months of total fasting. But, like Dick Gregory, you can live for a surprisingly long time on vegetable juices exclusively and be the better—and lighter—for it.

Removing Pesticides from Food

Real-world people shop at supermarkets, and real-world affordable fruits and vegetables contain pesticide residues. Not everybody can buy organic; not everybody is a gardener. Here are easy and effective ways to reduce your chemical consumption.

Rule number one: wash your fruits like you wash your hands: use soap! Mom was right: just running your mitts under tap water does little to remove oily grime. Agricultural pesticides do not come off in water, either. If they did, farmers would have to apply them after each rain or even a heavy dew. That would be both labor-intensive and expensive. So companies make pesticides with chemical "stickers" that are insoluble in water. They stay on the fruit, rain or shine.

Soap, or detergent, is more effective in removing pesticide residues than you think. You can prove this for yourself. Take a big bunch of red or green grapes, and place them, with a squirt of dishwashing detergent, in a large bowl of water. Mix the detergent in thoroughly, and swish the grapes around for a minute. Carefully watch the water. You will see evidence that detergent works. If you do not think that that stuff is pesticide residue, try another bowl of grapes in water without detergent, and try another bowl of organically grown grapes in water with detergent. Seeing is believing.

It is necessary to rinse detergent-washed fruits before eating, of course, but that is hardly a burden. Rinse until the water is clear. When you handle the detergent-washed fruit, you will also notice that it feels different, too. We are so used to fruit with chemical coatings that when we touch truly clean fruit, it's a new tactile experience. Go ahead, try it. Nobody's looking.

Even if you do not believe that pesticides pose the slightest health risk, there is no down side to not eating them. Whatever benefits they may confer on the tree, pesticides do you no good in your gut. Children may consume disproportionately large amounts of pesticides because kids eat a lot of fruit relative to their body weight. For parents, there is a measure of comfort in knowing that their kid's chemical intake has been minimized.

Newly detergent-washed fruit does not keep as well. The former petrochemical coating probably served as a moisture barrier and even an oxidation barrier (as does the wax coating on many fruits and vegetables). No worries; you only wash before you eat.

In case you think I am taking too easygoing a view of chemical farming, I would like to point out that I am an avid organic gardener. I also advocate purchasing organically grown foods whenever possible. It costs more to buy organic, but it is probably money well spent. Home gardening is an incredibly cheap alternative. All those stories that you hear about a thirty-dollar investment in seed and fertilizer yielding seven hundred dollars' worth of fresh food are true. If you think I'm more full of fertilizer than my garden is, I recommend that you try it and see. For starters, try leaf lettuce, zucchini, cucumbers, bush green beans, and a dozen tomato plants. You will soon be supplying half the neighborhood. None of these veggies require any pesticides to grow well.

A cheapskate hint: save those potatoes that are no good because they've sprouted eyes. The eyes are actually sprouts, each of which will grow into an entire potato plant bearing several spuds. Cut the tater up and plant each piece that has a sprout on it. No pesticides needed here, either.

Many fruits and vegetables are not merely sprayed, but are waxed as well. So-called "food grade" waxes improve shelf life and appearance, but also coat over and lock in any previously applied pesticides. This poses a problem, for waxes do not readily dissolve in detergent solution. You might find a product or two on the market that is certified to remove waxes from fruits, but the easiest alternative is simply to peel them. Frequently waxed produce includes apples, pears, eggplants, cucumbers, squash, and even tomatoes. The lack of a high gloss is not proof positive that a fruit is not waxed: many waxes, like many types of floor polyurethane or spray varnish, are not at all shiny. One way to tell if a fruit or vegetable is waxed is to run your fingernail over it and see if you can scrape anything off. Another way is to read the label and see if the produce is waxed. This may require a trip in back to the warehouse to see the carton that the produce came in. Lotsa luck on that.

A peeler costs under a buck and effectively removes wax. A squirt of dish detergent costs a few cents. Lots more information on pesticides is free and readily available on the Internet and from your public library.

214

Natural versus Synthetic Vitamins

Nobody really likes what I have to say on this subject. Vitamin salespeople think it's too medical, and medical people think it's too quacky. But facts are facts, and here are mine:

1. Most vitamin products sold in health-food stores contain synthetic vitamin powders. There are only a few manufacturers of vitamin powders, and they are generally large pharmaceutical companies. This is not an inherently bad thing, however, because laboratory-made vitamins are far cheaper than whole food concentrates, synthetic vitamins *usually* work quite well, and labs can get a significant potency into a small tablet.

   One of the biggest differences in "health-food store" versus "drug store" brands is what is *not* in the tablet. For example, most natural brands leave out artificial chemical colors, which is a good thing to do. Just about all brands contain tablet fillers and excipients, needed to physically hold the pill together. Since these will vary, the only way to find out exactly who uses what is to write to the company and ask. Some tableting ingredients are pretty standard: calcium-phosphate compounds, maltodextrin, silica or silicon dioxide, cellulose, and the stearates or stearic acid are common and widely accepted as harmless.

2. Vitamins can be called "natural" even if made in a laboratory. Vitamin C, for example, is factory-made from starch, which is a natural product. Is this starch-based vitamin C identical to orange-juice-based vitamin C? Most biochemists say yes. But the real test is effectiveness. High doses of factory-made ascorbic acid vitamin C work against viral and bacterial illness, and in numerous other illnesses. It is possible that food-concentrate vitamin C may be somewhat more efficient, but because it would be so much more expensive, it isn't worth it.

3. In some cases, however, the natural form of a vitamin *is* clearly superior to the synthetic form. The best example is vitamin E. The natural form of vitamin E is called "D-alpha-tocopherol," and is derived from vegetable oil. The petrochemically based synthetic form is DL-alpha-tocopherol. Not a big difference in name, is it? But there

215

is considerable evidence that the natural form of vitamin E is more useful to the body than is the synthetic. The natural form is also more expensive, but not that much more. In choosing a vitamin E supplement, you should always look for D-alpha-tocopherol. It is even better if the product contains additional vitamin E cofactors usually called "mixed natural tocopherols."

It is remarkable how many natural-looking brown bottles, with naturally decorated labels and natural-sounding brand names, contain the synthetic form. I once bought just such an innocent-looking package, only to discover that the pills inside were a dazzling, nearly radioactive pink color. Strange, but true. I still have them, and I like to trot them out during lectures as proof.

216

Ten Ways to Spot Antivitamin Biases in a Scientific Study

1. Where's the beef? How much of the original study is quoted in the media? Are you just getting factoids, or are data provided? Has the journalist writing about the subject read the original paper?

2. What exactly was studied, and how? Was it an *in vitro* (test tube) study or an *in vivo* (animal) study? Was there a *clinical study* on people, or is its application to real life a matter of conjecture?

3. Follow the money. Who paid for the study? Cash from food processors, pharmaceutical giants, and other deep pockets decides what gets studied, and how. It is very difficult, if not impossible, for researchers to present findings that embarrass their financial backers. Published research will often indicate sources of funding, possibly at the end of the paper in an acknowledgments paragraph. If not, correspondence addresses of principal authors are invariably provided. Write and ask.

4. Check the dosages. Any vitamin C study using less than 2,000 mg a day is a waste of time. Any vitamin E study employing less than 400 IU is a waste of time. Any niacin study using less than 1,000 mg a day is a waste of time.

5. Check the form of supplement used. Was the vitamin used in the study natural or synthetic? Any carotene study using the synthetic form of beta-carotene only is useless. Any vitamin E study using the synthetic DL-alpha-tocopherol form is useless.

6. Use the "Pauling Principle": read the entire study and interpret the data for yourself. Do not rely on the summary or conclusions of the authors. As Linus Pauling pointed out repeatedly, many researchers miss, or dismiss, the statistical significance of their own work. Such behavior may be human error, or it may be politically motivated. Beware of editorializing.

7. Beware of Pauling-bashers. If a media article is critical about Nobel prize–winning Linus Pauling, you can be sure it has been spin-doctored.

8. Watch for assumptions from the authors that we get all the vitamins we need from diet, or that there is no scientific support for large vitamin doses.

9. Watch for ultra-cautious public recommendations at the end of the article such as "Just eat a balanced diet" or "If you must take vitamins, take no more than the RDA."

10. Use the media backwards. The more headlines about a particular study, the more politically charged the subject and the less likely that the reporting, or the original study, is objective. Positive new drug studies get headlines. So do vitamin scare stories. The more media hoopla, the worse the research. Truly valuable research does not scare people; it helps people get well.

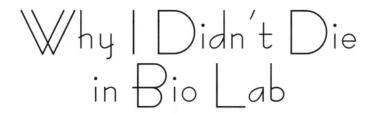

Why I Didn't Die in Bio Lab

The germ is nothing; the terrain is everything.
LOUIS PASTEUR

Let me tell you about the kid who was my lab partner in high school biology class, and who was always, always sick. Mike came to class hacking on what seemed to be an everyday basis. Naturally, his assigned seat was right next to me, at the shiny black-topped table-for-two that was so common in science classrooms. All through lectures, he sniffed, snorted, and sneezed. All through lab, he hacked, coughed, and gagged. This kid was sickly. You've got to give him high marks for showing up at all, but he had annoyingly good attendance, which was just my luck.

One day we were doing agar culture plates. This means you mix up some diarrhea-colored, Jell-O-like stuff, heat it, and pour it into shallow, round, four-inch-diameter glass dishes. After it cools, you add some bacteria or whatever microorganism you wish to grow. We'd stocked the incubator with a nice variety of specimens, and had a few extra, unused culture plates all dressed up with nowhere to go.

The lab manual said to leave one out in the classroom, uncovered, and see if a culture could be obtained from what settled out from the air. We went it one better.

We used Mike.

Almost at the same moment, we all came to the realization that Mike was our local one-stop source of pathogens. And, Mr. Thorensen being out of the room at that particular moment, our chance had come. We had Mike cough all over a couple of agar plates. I mean, he really let it all out. The girls turned away into their handkerchiefs. The boys grimaced and kept watching, wincing when a really shattering blast erupted from Mike's capacious lungs.

As Mike was mopping up the table in front of him, we light-footed it to the rear of the lab, covered our extracurricular cultures, and stuck them in the incubator, on the bottom shelf, way in the back. Visions of a Nobel dancing in our heads, we zipped back to our seats just as Mr. Thorensen walked in. We gave him our best cheesy smiles and folded our hands to await his next pronouncement, or the bell, whichever came first.

219

Naturally, we completely forgot about those culture plates. They were unlabeled, so nobody claimed them, but nobody threw them out, either.

Considerable time went by.

When Mr. Thorensen was out of the room again one day, we recalled our impromptu research project. My pal Sid and I went back to the old gray incubator, opened it, and reached all the way in. Ah yes, there they were, still. We brought the two dishes out and everyone gathered around to see some real science.

It was just gorgeous. Big, hairy black growths, white puffballs, and layers of milky slime covered the culture surface. Ugh. It looked like you'd exhumed the guts of a rotting carp. Gross. Then and there, we knew two things. First: Mike should, by all logic, be dead. Second: all too obviously, he wasn't.

Being Mike's closest friend, in a geographical sense, I had a personal stake in this. I should, at the very least, have had Mike's symptoms in spades.

But I didn't. Somehow, my body was keeping me healthy, in the face of the worst that Mike's propagated population of pathogens could do.

My life in natural healing began that very moment. Pasteur was right: it's not the seed; it's the soil. You can cough on a steel plate and the culture will fail to thrive. If your body gets what it needs, it will stay healthy, no matter what lurks in the lungs of your neighbor.

A Crash Course in Vegetarian Cooking

When I was a kid, eating was a necessary evil. Mom, a former history teacher, did not exactly have a passion for cooking. Her casual disregard of any advances ever made in culinary science approached the legendary. Years ago, my daughter based an essay for English class on the time in my boyhood when my mother mixed a box of lime Jell-O with a box of cherry Jell-O and got gray Jell-O. Yes, we had to eat it. You didn't waste food in our home.

"Well done," at least in my experience, is the ultimate oxymoron. Mom could have burned ice cream. She overcooked everything, justifying it with the ever-ready apology, "Your father likes it this way." After years and years of eating overdone, dry, tooth-stressing meals, I finally asked Pop why he liked everything overcooked. He said, "That's the way your mother makes it." O. Henry would have been pleased.

Perhaps it was this palate-punishing perversion of what should have been home cooking that sent me running in the other direction as an adult. Whatever it was, I've been cooking with whole, natural, vegetarian foods for thirty years now. Here are my ten best kitchen tips. (Remember, however, that you are getting these suggestions from a guy who, as a college graduate, still thought allspice was a mixture of all the spices together in one convenient jar.)

1. If there is one secret of vegetarian cooking, it is salt. Grains and legumes (peas, beans, and lentils) especially need it for good taste. Now don't go worrying that you are getting too much sodium. Homemade foods have less salt than most store-bought processed foods, and certainly are less salty than restaurant foods. Use (just) enough salt to make people want to eat what you serve, and you have won half the battle. If you overdo it, too much salt can be removed from food by cooking a halved raw potato into your mistake and then removing the potato before serving. Adding more water, or more of all the other ingredients, will also reduce the salt concentration.

2. Taste your cooking as you go. If you like it, others probably will. Learning from mistakes is less costly if you own a nice, hungry, tolerant doggie. Such animals are readily available from your local pound or humane society. Believe me, anything

you were previously thinking of tossing out is far better than the stuff that goes into most commercial pet foods.

3. Consult easy vegetarian cookbooks. I especially like *The Deaf Smith Country Cookbook* and *Laurel's Kitchen.* Health food stores tend to have a good selection of cookbooks, and often have free recipes for the asking.

4. When in doubt, leave it out. If you are not sure whether to use an ingredient, don't. I've made bread with just whole wheat flour, water, and salt. Period. It yields a flatbread or Johnnycake, but it tastes great. I never add shortening or oil to my raised breads; you really don't miss it.

5. Over the years, you will save a fortune cooking vegetarian. (Just don't make your fortune cooking vegetarians, which is illegal.) The best foods in the supermarket are often the cheapest; the worst foods cost the most. We spend only about one third as much on food as our neighbors do. We have here a way to make money getting healthy. Can you beat that?

6. Start small, but when you get experienced try to cook in quantity. A big pot of soup will feed you all week. Keep it in meal-sized containers in your refrigerator. Open one of those instead of a can of something. Just as convenient, but cheaper and healthier, too.

7. Be sure to cook beans and dry legumes thoroughly. They taste dreadful if you don't. After checking to remove any little stowaway stones, soak your legumes tonight to reduce cooking time tomorrow. Change the soaking water twice before cooking to remove dirt or soap residues.

8. If you are not used to baking with whole wheat flour, work it in gradually. Start with $2/3$ white (unbleached) flour and $1/3$ whole wheat. Then try half and half. Over time, you can increase the fraction of whole wheat so subtly that no one will notice. Baking with all whole wheat (or any other whole grain) generally requires more leavening and more cooking time. Pull up a chair by the oven and check from time to time.

9. To stimulate your cooking habit, keep *less* food in the house. The more convenience crutches we have, the less we work at self-reliance. Stock up on grains and legumes. Being dry, they keep a long time in glass jars or plastic bags. With salt, oil, some herbs and spices, and of course fruits and vegetables, you are set. Butter, cheese, and yogurt are part of our menu, but need not be for some. Tofu, tempeh, sprouts or seed for sprouting, honey, molasses, and fruit juice fill out our cheap diet. We are most creative in the kitchen when the pickings are slim.

10. Do not fret if you succumb to a Big Mac Attack or wolf down the occasional box of chocolates. To me, it is not a matter of life or death if you have turkey at the hol-

222

idays (though it is to the turkey). What matters is not what you do on any one day but what you do on the other 364. In total, are you doing it right? Check your debts; check your medicine cabinet use; check the bathroom scales: if they are all going down, you are doing fine.

AFTERWORD:
It's Your Decision, Your Health, Your Life

The whole idea of doctoring yourself is to promote health self-reliance. I like to call it "health homesteading." This is easy talk when you are well, but admittedly a tougher row to hoe when you are sick. As I've stressed throughout this book, it is vital to have reliable information at hand so that you can confidently make decisions about your family's health. Here are some real ways to get detailed, accurate answers to your health questions. All require a measure of personal commitment:

1. Do a search at your local public library, and ask your librarian for assistance. Your library cannot possibly be smaller than the two-room Hamlin Public Library I use in upstate New York, and even out here we have five computer terminals and some of the most helpful librarians I've seen anywhere (and I've met a lot of librarians in my time). This will cost you no money at all.

2. Do a thorough search on the Internet, using several major search engines. In the age of computers, it is easier than ever to quickly mine the vaults of learning. But it helps to know where to do the digging. Give a hungry person a fish and he will be hungry again tomorrow. Teach a person how to fish, and he will always have food. Do not stop at only one or two websites; check them all. The following cautions apply:

   Beware of websites that have a product for sale. Such sites will not be objective. You may have to look very carefully to find the product affiliation within a website, but it is worth the search.

   Beware of so-called consumer-protection sites warning of the dangers of vitamin use. Such misinformation is fifty years out of date. If a site tells you *not* to read something, you should make a point to go and read it immediately.

   Be cautious of sites run by private physicians or other individuals who make their money through consultation services. Such professionals have an interest in offering you some promising free information, and then charging you for the real service.

   For that matter, be cautious of *any* site run by *anyone.* This includes my own website, DoctorYourself.com. Use my CELERY system: **C**heck **E**very **L**iterature reference and personal **E**xperience, and **R**ead for **Y**ourself.

If this all sounds like work, well, of course it is. Life is work. You have to eat anyway; you might as well eat right. You have to spend time on your health; better the library than the doctor's waiting room. Consider the actual time-saving benefits: improving your health will pay you back, not only with more years of life but better years of life. If this is too much for you, then you are ready to die. If you are not ready to die, learn to love libraries, bibliographies, and reading. If I gave your topic of interest short shrift in this book, you can be sure that the library and the Internet do not.

As a health consultant, I am daily inundated with people wanting to skip the time-consuming research steps outlined above and instead ask me, in passing, what to do for their health problem. It is called "curbside advice," and I can't blame them for trying. Still, it takes no time at all to formulate the question: "What should I do for so-and-so?" Now, after years of deliberation, I finally have what may be the closest thing to a concise answer:

You need to change your entire life.

Change your life. If you want to get better, that is what you have to do. The first step is to read a lot, a whole lot. But that is only the beginning.

If you've never tried being a vegetarian, start.

If you've never juiced vegetables, start.

If you've never read the *Journal of Orthomolecular Medicine,* start.

If you've never taken vitamin C to saturation, start.

If you've never taught your doctor something, start.

If you've never taken a course in how to meditate or otherwise reduce stress, start.

If you've never done a half-hour fitness workout each day, start.

If you've never given up alcohol or smoking, start. (No, wise guy, I don't mean start smoking!)

If you've never used an interlibrary loan to get a valuable health book, start.

If these things sound impossible to you, then what are you asking the question for? If you have already limited your response, why inquire at all?

To quickly cut through the treacle, I ask clients this most pointed of questions early in a consultation: "What are you willing to do to get better?" The answer I want, of course, is, "Anything." But as with New Year's resolutions, I know better than to hold people too rigorously to their dreams. Flexibility was never more necessary than with self-health care. I will accept a two-thirds effort, for, as a teacher of some experience, I pass anyone at a grade of 65. More is better, but if you were to entirely change two-thirds of your life, I'd be satisfied and impressed. Especially if you held to it for more than a year.

I think you'd be even more impressed with the results.

I see two kinds of sick people: those that do not want to change their lifestyle, and those that do, but don't know where to start. Prospecting for gold and seeking better health are similar in three ways:

1. You need the motivation to get rich.

2. You need information on where to dig.

3. You need to do the digging.

There is no such thing as a free lunch, a quick fix, or a magic wand to cure illness. I wish there were easy answers to people's health questions. There aren't. There are answers, all right, but they are not easy. Modern medicine has created more codependents even than copays. We've learned to hold out for the magic bullet, the new miracle drug, the breakthrough surgical procedure. We've also "learned" to discount the healing power of nature, and the tremendous therapeutic benefit of lifestyle changes, vegetarian diet, raw food juices, and vitamin supplements.

But times are changing. There is a new paradigm, an entirely new way of seeing health, opening in front of us. You may have heard that the Chinese word for "crisis" is the same as the word for "opportunity." There, in a nutshell, lies the *Doctor Yourself* philosophy. Whatever opportunity you are looking for, you must follow leads and dig. Whether it is for oil, gold, information, or health, it requires action. Your action. If you want to change your health, you have to change your life. Do it today.

Bibliography

Adams R and Murray F. *Megavitamin Therapy.* New York: Larchmont, 1973.

Airola P. *Health Secrets from Europe.* New York: Arco, 1972.

Airola P. *How to Get Well.* Phoenix, AZ: Health Plus, 1980.

Bailey H. *The Vitamin Pioneers.* Emmaus, PA: Rodale Books, 1968.

Bailey H. *Vitamin E for a Healthy Heart and a Longer Life.* New York: Carroll and Graf, 1993.

Balch J and Balch P. *Prescription for Nutritional Healing.* Garden City Park, NY: Avery, 1990.

Barnett LB. New concepts in bone healing. *Journal of Applied Nutrition* 7 (1954): 318–23.

Belfield WO. Vitamin C in treatment of canine and feline distemper complex. *Veterinary Medicine/Small Animal Clinician* (April 1967): 345–48.

Bernier RH, et al. Diphtheria-tetanus toxoids-pertussis vaccination and sudden infant deaths in Tennessee. *Jour Pediatrics* 101 (1982): 419–21.

Bicknell F and Prescott F. *The Vitamins in Medicine,* 3rd ed. Milwaukee, WI: Lee Foundation, 1953.

Billings E and Westmore A. *The Billings Method.* New York: Ballantine, 1983.

Bircher R. "A Turning Point in Nutritional Science." Address delivered in Milwaukee, WI, c. 1950. Undated reprint by Lee Foundation for Nutritional Research, Milwaukee, WI.

Bland J. *The Key to the Power of Vitamin C and Its Metabolites.* New Canaan, CT: Keats Publishing, 1989.

Block G, et al. Epidemiological evidence regarding vitamin C and cancer. *American Journal of Clinical Nutrition* 54 (December 1991): 1310S– 314S.

Burgstahler A. Water fluoridation: promise and reality. *National Fluoridation News* (Summer 1985).

Burns D, ed. *The Greatest Health Discovery: Natural Hygiene and Its Evolution, Past Present and Future.* Chicago: Natural Hygiene Press, 1972.

Cameron E. Vitamin C and cancer: an overview. *International Journal of Vitamin and Nutrition Research* Suppl. 23 (1982): 115–127.

Cameron E. "Protocol for the Use of Intravenous Vitamin C in the Treatment of Cancer." Palo Alto, CA: Linus Pauling Institute of Science and Medicine, undated.

Cameron E. Protocol for the use of vitamin C in the treatment of cancer. *Medical Hypotheses* 36 (1991): 190–94.

Cameron E and Baird G. Ascorbic acid and dependence on opiates in patients with advanced and disseminated cancer. *Journal of International Research Communications* 1 (1973): 38.

Cameron E and Campbell A. The orthomolecular treatment of cancer II. Clinical trial of high-dose ascorbic supplements in advanced human cancer. *Chemical-Biological Interactions* 9 (1974): 285–315.

Cameron E and Campbell A. Innovation vs. quality control: an "unpublishable" clinical trial of supplemental ascorbate in incurable cancer. *Medical Hypotheses* 36 (1991): 185–189.

Cameron E and Pauling L. Ascorbic acid and the glycosaminoglycans: An orthomolecular approach to cancer and other diseases. *Oncology* (Basel) 27 (1973): 181–192.

Cameron E and Pauling L. The orthomolecular treatment of cancer. 1. The role of ascorbate in host resistance. *Chemical-Biological Interactions* 9 (1974): 273–83.

Cameron E and Pauling L. Supplemental ascorbate in the supportive treatment of cancer: prolongation of survival times in terminal human cancer. *Proceedings of the National Academy of Sciences USA* 73 (1976): 3685–689.

Cameron E and Pauling L. Supplemental ascorbate in the supportive treatment of cancer: Reevaluation of prolongation of survival times in terminal human cancer. *Proceed-*

ings of the National Academy of Sciences USA 75 (1978): 4538–542.

Cameron E and Pauling L. *Cancer and Vitamin C,* revised edition. Philadelphia: Camino Books, 1993.

Campbell A, Jack T, and Cameron E. Reticulum cell sarcoma: two complete "spontanous" regressions, in response to high-dose ascorbic acid therapy. A report on subsequent progress. *Oncology* 48 (1991): 495–97.

Canter L. *Assertive Discipline for Parents,* revised edition. New York: Harper and Row, 1985.

Carnegie D. *How to Win Friends and Influence People.* New York: Pocket Books, 1981.

Carper J. *Food: Your Miracle Medicine.* New York: Harper-Collins, 1993.

Carter CW. Maintenance nutrition in the pigeon and its relation to heart block. *Biochemistry* 28 (1934): 933–39.

Cathcart RF. Clinical trial of vitamin C. [Letter to the editor.] *Medical Tribune* (25 June 1975).

Cathcart RF. The method of determining proper doses of vitamin C for the treatment of disease by titrating to bowel tolerance. *Journal of Orthomolecular Psychiatry* 10 (1981): 125–132.

Cathcart RF. Titration to bowel tolerance, anascorbemia, and acute induced scurvy. *Medical Hypotheses* 7 (1981): 1359–376.

Cathcart RF. Vitamin C in the treatment of acquired immune deficiency syndrome (AIDS). *Medical Hypotheses* 14 (1984): 423–33.

Cathcart RF. Vitamin C, the nontoxic, nonrate-limited antioxidant free radical scavenger. *Medical Hypotheses* 18 (1985): 61–77.

Cathcart RF. The vitamin C treatment of allergy and the normally unprimed state of antibodies. *Medical Hypotheses* 21 (1986): 307–21.

Cathcart RF. A unique function for ascorbate. *Medical Hypotheses* 35 (May 1991): 32–37.

Cathcart RF. The third face of vitamin C. *Journal of Orthomolecular Medicine* 7 (1993): 197–200.

Chakrabarti RN and Dasgupta PS. Effects of ascorbic acid on survival and cell-mediated immunity in tumor bearing mice. *IRCS Med Sci* 12 (1984): 1147–148.

Challem J. *Vitamin C Updated.* New Canaan, CT: Keats Publishing, 1983.

Chan AC. Vitamin E and atherosclerosis.[Review.] *J Nutr* 128 (October 1998): 1593–596.

Chapman-Smith D. Cost effectiveness: the Manga report. *The Chiropractic Report* (1993): 1–2.

Cheney G. Rapid healing of peptic ulcers in patients receiving fresh cabbage juice. *California Medicine* 70 (1949): 10–14.

Cheney G. Anti-peptic ulcer dietary factor. *J Am Diet Assoc* 26 (1950): 668–72.

Cheney, G. Vitamin U therapy of peptic ulcer. *California Medicine* 77 (1952): 248–52.

Cheraskin E and Ringsdorf WM. *New Hope for Incurable Diseases.* New York: Exposition Press, 1971.

Cheraskin E, et al. *The Vitamin C Connection.* New York: Harper and Row, 1983.

Chopra D. *Perfect Health.* New York: Harmony Books, 1991.

Clarke JH. *The Prescriber.* Essex, England: CW Daniel, 1972.

Cleave TL. *The Saccharine Disease.* New Canaan, CT: Keats Publishing, 1974.

Cleigh Z. Laetrile. *Well Being Magazine* 26 (November 1977): 29–33.

Coulter H. *Homeopathic Influences in Nineteenth-Century Allopathic Therapeutics.* Falls Church VA: American Institute of Homeopathy, 1973.

Coulter H. *Homoeopathic Science and Modern Medicine.* Richmond, CA: North Atlantic Books, 1981.

Coulter H and Fisher B. *A Shot in the Dark.* Garden City Park, NY: Avery, 1991.

Cowley G. Healer of hearts. *Newsweek* (16 March 1998): 50–56.

Cumming F. Vaccinations: A health hazard? *Sydney Sunday Herald* (4 April 1993): 41–42, 79.

Dahl H and Degre M. The effect of ascorbic acid on production of human interferon and the antiviral activity in vitro. *Acta Pathologica et Microbiologica Scandinavica* 84 (1976): 280–84.

Dannenburg AM, et al. Ascorbic acid in the treatment of chronic lead poisoning. *JAMA* 114 (1940): 1439–440.

Davis A. *Let's Get Well.* New York: Signet, 1965.

Davis A. *Let's Eat Right to Keep Fit.* New York: Signet, 1970.

Dawson EB, et al. Effects of ascorbic acid on male fertility. In "Third Conference on Vitamin C," *Annals of the New York Academy of Sciences* 498 (1987).

Dawson W and West GB. The influence of ascorbic acid on histamine metabolism in guinea pigs. *British Journal of Pharmacology* 24 (1965): 725–34.

Dufty W. *Sugar Blues.* New York: Warner Books, 1975.

Dworkin S and Dworkin F. *The Apartment Gardener.* New York: Signet, 1974.

Dworkin S and Dworkin F. *The Good Goodies.* New York: Fawcett Crest, 1974.

Eby G, Davis D, and Halcomb W. Reduction in duration of common cold symptoms by zinc gluconate lozenges in a double blind study. *Antimicrobal Agents and Chemotherapy* 25 (January 1984): 20–24.

Edward JF. Iodine: its use in the treatment and prevention of poliomyelitis and allied diseases. *Manitoba Medical Review* 34 (1954): 337–39.

Enstrom JE, Kanim LE, and Klein MA. Vitamin C intake and mortality among a sample of the United States population. *Epidemiology* 3 (1992): 194–202.

Fairfield KM and Fletcher RH. Vitamins for Chronic Disease Prevention in Adults: Scientific Review. *JAMA.* 2002; 287:3116-3126.

Farrell W. *Why Men Are the Way They Are.* New York: McGraw-Hill, 1986.

Farrell W. *The Myth of Male Power.* New York: Simon and Schuster, 1993.

Feingold BF. *Why Your Child is Hyperactive.* New York: Random House, 1985.

Fletcher RH and Fairfield KM. Vitamins for Chronic Disease Prevention in Adults: Clinical Applications. *JAMA.* 2002; 287:3127-3129.

Ford MW, et al. *The Deaf Smith Country Cookbook.* New York: Collier, 1973.

Fredericks C and Bailey H. *Food Facts and Fallacies.* New York: Arco, 1965.

Free V and Sanders P. The use of ascorbic acid and mineral supplements in the detoxification of narcotic addicts. *Journal of Orthomolecular Psychiatry* 7 (1978): 264–70.

Fritsch A and The Center for Science in the Public Interest. *99 Ways to a Simple Lifestyle.* New York: Anchor-Doubleday, 1977.

Furgurson EB. *Chancellorsville, 1863.* New York: Alfred A. Knopf, 1992.

Gerson M. *A Cancer Therapy: Results of Fifty Cases,* 3rd ed. Del Mar, CA: Totality Books, 1977.

Gerson C and Walker M. *The Gerson Therapy.* New York: Kensington Publishing Corp, 2001.

Ghosh J and Das S. Evaluation of vitamin A and C status in normal and malignant conditions and their possible role in cancer prevention. *Japanese Journal of Cancer Research* 76 (December 1995): 1174–178.

Goldbeck N and Goldbeck D. *The Supermarket Handbook.* New York: Signet, 1976.

Goodman S. *Vitamin C: The Master Nutrient.* New Canaan, CT: Keats Publishing, 1991.

Graves SB. Carrots and cancer: the surprising connection. *Family Circle* (1 July 1982).

Greenwood J. Optimum vitamin C intake as a factor in the preservation of disk integrity. *Med Ann DC.* 33 (June 1964).

Gregory D. *Dick Gregory's Natural Diet for Folks Who Eat.* New York: Harper and Row, 1973.

Griffin MR, et al. Risk of sudden infant death syndrome after immunization with the diphtheria-tetanus-pertussis vaccine. *New Engl Jour Med* 319 (1988): 618–23.

Gross L. The effects of vitamin deficient diets on rats, with special reference to the motor functions of the intestinal tract in vivo and in vitro. *Journal of Pathology and Bacteriology* 27 (1924): 27–50.

Growdon A. "Neurotransmitter Precursors in the Diet." In *Nutrition and the Brain,* edited by Wurtman and Wurtman. New York: Raven Press, 1979, 117–81.

Guenther RM. Alcoholism and nutrition. *International Journal of Biosocial Research* 4 (1983): 3–4.

Harrell RF, et al. Can nutritional supplements help mentally retarded children? An exploratory study. *Proceedings of the National Academy of Sciences USA* 78 (1981): 574–78.

Harris A, Robinson A, and Pauling L. Blood plasma l-ascorbic acid concentration for oral l-ascorbic acid dosage up to 12 grams per day. *International Research Communications System* (December 1973): 19.

Hart BF and Levensdorf M. Is there an alternative to surgery for angina pectoris? *Let's Live* (October 1977).

Hawkins DR, Bortin AW, Runyon RP. Orthomolecular psychiatry: niacin and megavitamin therapy. *Psychosomatics* 11(1970): 517–21.

Hawkins DR and Pauling L. *Orthomolecular Psychiatry.* San Francisco: Freeman, 1973.

Hemil H. Vitamin C and the common cold. *British Journal of Nutrition* 67 (1992): 3–16.

Hillemann HH. The illusion of American health and longevity. *Clinical Physiology* 2 (1960): 120–77.

Hoffer A. "Relation of Epinephrine Metabolites to Schizophrenia." In *Chemical Concepts of Psychiatry,* edited by M Rinkel and HGB Denber. New York: Mowell-Obolensky Inc, 1958.

Hoffer A. *Niacin Therapy in Psychiatry.* Springfield, IL: Charles S. Thomas, 1962.

Hoffer A. Treatment of schizophrenia. *Orthomolecular Psychiatry* 3 (1974): 280–90.

Hoffer A. *Vitamin B_3 and Schizophrenia: Discovery, Recovery, Controversy.* Kingston, ON: Quarry Press, 1998.

Hoffer A. *Dr. Hoffer's ABC of Natural Nutrition for Children.* Kingston, ON: Quarry Press, 1999.

Hoffer A. *Vitamin C and Cancer: Discovery, Recovery, Controversy.* Kingston, ON: Quarry Press, 1999.

Hoffer A and Osmond H. Treatment of schizophrenia with nicotinic acid: a ten-year follow-up. *Acta Psychiatr Scand* 40 (1964): 171–89.

Hoffer A and Osmond H. *New Hope for Alcoholics.* New Hyde Park, NY: University Books, 1968.

Hoffer A, Osmond H, Callbeck JM, and Kahan I. Treatment of schizophrenia with nicotinic acid and nicotinamide. *Journal of Clinical Experimental Psychopathology* 18 (1957): 131–58.

Hoffer A and Pauling L. Hardin Jones biostatistical analysis of mortality data for cohorts of cancer patients with a large fraction surviving at the termination of the study and a comparison of survival times of cancer patients receiving large regular oral doses of vitamin C and other nutrients with similar patients not receiving those doses. *Journal of Orthomolecular Medicine* 5 (1990): 143–54.

Hoffer A and Pauling L. Hardin Jones biostatistical analysis of mortality data for a second set of cohorts of cancer patients with a large fraction surviving at the termination of the study and a comparison of survival times of cancer patients receiving large regular oral doses of vitamin C and other nutrients with similar patients not receiving those doses. *Journal of Orthomolecular Medicine* 8 (1993): 157–67.

Hoffmann-La Roche. "Marginal Vitamin Deficiency: The Gray Area of Nutrition." [Reprint.] La Canada, CA: Bronson Pharmaceuticals, (undated brochure).

Horwitt MK. Vitamin E: a reexamination. *American Journal of Clinical Nutrition* 29 (5 May 1976).

Horwitz N. Vitamins, minerals boost IQ in retarded. *Medical Tribune* 22 (1981): 1, 19.

Huggins H. *It's All in Your Head. Diseases Caused by Silver-Mercury Fillings.* Colorado Springs, CO: Life Sciences Press, 1990.

Hume ED. *Bechamp or Pasteur? A Lost Chapter in the History of Biology.* London: C.W. Daniel, 1923.

Humer RP. Brain food: Neurotransmitters make you think. *Let's Live* (December 1981).

Hunter BT. *The Natural Foods Cookbook.* New York: Pyramid, 1961.

Hutton E. The fight over vitamin E. *Maclean's Magazine* (15 June 1953).

Illich I. *Deschooling Society.* New York: Harper and Row, 1970.

Illich I. *Medical Nemesis.* New York: Bantam, 1976.

Inglis B. *The Case for Unorthodox Medicine.* New York: Putnam, 1965.

Issac K and Gold S, ed. *Eating Clean 2: Overcoming Food Hazards.* Washington, DC: Center for Study of Responsive Law, 1987.

Jarvis DC. *Folk Medicine.* New York: Holt, 1958.

Johnston EA. Vitamins and their relation to diseases of the alimentary tract. *Journal of the American College of Proctology* [Undated reprint].

Jungeblut CW. Inactivation of poliomyelitis virus by crystallin vitamin C (ascorbic acid). *Journal of Experimental Medicine* 62 (1935): 517–21.

Jungeblut CW. Further observations on vitamin C therapy in experimental poliomyelitis. *Journal of Experimental Medicine* 65 (1939): 127–46.

Jungeblut CW. A further contribution to the vitamin C therapy in experimental poliomyelitis. *Journal of Experimental Medicine* 70 (1939): 327.

Kalokerinos A. *Every Second Child.* New Canaan, CT: Keats Publishing, 1981.

Kaufman W. *Common Forms of Niacinamide Deficiency Disease: Aniacin Amidosis.* New Haven, CT: Yale University Press, 1943.

Kaufman W. *The Common Form of Joint Dysfunction: Its Incidence and Treatment.* Brattleboro, VT: E. L. Hildreth and Co., 1949.

Kirschner HE. Comfrey. *Let's Live* (October–December 1958).

Klenner FR. Treating multiple sclerosis nutritionally. *Cancer Control Journal* 2 (3): 16–20 [Undated].

Klenner FR. Virus pneumonia and its treatment with vitamin C. *Southern Medicine and Surgery* 110 (February 1948): 36–38, 46.

Klenner FR. The treatment of poliomyelitis and other virus diseases with vitamin C. *Southern Medicine and Surgery* 113 (1949): 101–107.

Klenner FR. Massive doses of vitamin C and the virus diseases. *Southern Medicine and Surgery* 103 (1951): 101–07.

Klenner FR. The use of vitamin C as an antibiotic. *Journal of Applied Nutrition* 6 (1953): 274–78.

Klenner FR. The history of lockjaw. *Tri-State Medical Journal* (June 1954).

Klenner FR. Recent discoveries in the treatment of lockjaw. *Tri-State Medical Journal* (July 1954).

Klenner FR. The role of ascorbic acid in therapeutics. *Tri-State Medical Journal* (November 1955).

Klenner FR. Observations on the dose of administration of ascorbic acid when employed beyond the range of a vitamin in human pathology. *Journal of Applied Nutrition* 23 (Winter 1971): 61–68.

Klenner FR. Response of peripheral and central nerve pathology to megadoses of the vitamin B complex and other metabolites. *Journal of Applied Nutrition* 25 (1973): 16.

Klenner FR. "Significance of High Daily Intake of Ascorbic Acid in Preventive Medicine." In *A Physician's Handbook on Orthomolecular Medicine,* edited by RJ Williams and DK Kalita. New Canaan, CT: Keats Publishing, 1979.

Kordish J. *The Juiceman's Power of Juicing.* New York: William Morrow, 1992.

Kulvinskas V. *Survival into the 21st Century.* Wethersfield, CT: Omangod Press, 1975.

Landrigan PJ and Witte JJ. Neurologic disorders following live measles-virus vaccination. *JAMA* 223 (1973): 1459–62.

Lasagna L. One-a-day, plus C. *The Sciences* (November 1981), 35.

Lasky MS. *The Complete Junk Food Book.* New York: McGraw-Hill, 1977.

Law D. *A Guide to Alternative Medicine.* Garden City, NY: Dolphin, 1976.

Lee R. *Clinical Nutrition: Food vs. Drugs.* Milwaukee, WI: Lee Foundation for Nutritional Research, [undated].

Lee R. Vitamins in dental care. *Health Culture* (May 1955).

Levin M and Hartzell W. Ascorbic acid: the concept of optimum requirements. In "Third Conference on Vitamin C," *Annals of the New York Academy of Sciences* 498: (1987).

Levy T. *Vitamin C, Infectious Diseases, and Toxins: Curing the Incurable.* Philadelphia, PA: Xlibris, 2002.

Lewin S. *Vitamin C: Its Molecular Biology and Medical Potential.* London: Academic Press, 1976.

Lin D. Extensive clinical uses of vitamin E. *Nutritional Perspectives* (July 1992): 16–28.

Abrupt termination of high daily intake of vitamin C: the rebound effect. *Linus Pauling Institute of Science and Medicine Newsletter* 2 (1985): 6.

Loeffler W. Department of Education and Human Development Lecture. State University College at Brockport, New York (3 November 1986).

Lupulescu A. The role of vitamins A, beta-carotene, E and C in cancer cell biology. *International Journal of Vitamin and Nutrition Research* 64 (1994): 3–14.

Lust JB. *The Herb Book.* New York: Bantam, 1974.

MacAlister CJ and Titherley AW. *Narrative of an Investigation Concerning an Ancient Medicinal Remedy and its Modern Utilities Together with an Account of the Chemical Constitution of Allantoin.* London: John Bale, Sons, and Danielsson, 1936.

Machlin LJ. Beyond deficiency: new views on the function and health effects of vitamins. [Introduction.] *Annals of the New York Academy of Sciences* 669 (1992): 1–6.

Massell BE, Warren JE, Patterson PR, et al. Antirheumatic activity of ascorbic acid in large doses. *New England Journal of Medicine* (1950).

McCormick WJ. Lithogenesis and hypovitaminosis. *Medical Record* 159 (July 1946).

McCormick WJ. The changing incidence and mortality of infectious disease in relation to changed trends in nutrition. *Medical Record* (September 1947).

McCormick WJ. Ascorbic acid as a chemotherapeutic agent. Archives of Pediatrics of New York 69 (April 1952): 151–55.

McCormick WJ. Coronary thrombosis: the number one killer. *Insurance Index* (May 1953): 88–91.

McCormick WJ. Cancer: The preconditioning factor in pathogenesis. *Archives of Pediatrics of New York* 71 (1954): 313.

McCormick WJ. Intervertebral disc lesions: a new etiological concept. *Archives of Pediatrics of New York* 71 (1954): 29–33.

McCormick WJ. Coronary thrombosis: a new concept of mechanism and etiology. *Clinical Medicine* 4 (July 1957).

McCormick WJ. Have we forgotten the lesson of scurvy? *Journal of Applied Nutrition* 15 (1962): 4–12.

Meares A. *Relief without Drugs.* London: Souvenir Press, 1994.

Mendelsohn RS. *Confessions of a Medical Heretic.* Chicago: Contemporary Books, 1979.

Mendelsohn RS. *How to Raise a Healthy Child in Spite of Your Doctor.* New York: Ballantine Books, 1985.

Miller NZ. Vaccines and natural health. *Mothering* (Spring 1994): 44–54.

Miller NZ. *Immunization: Theory vs. Reality—Expose on Vaccinations.* Santa Fe, NM: New Atlantean Press, 1996.

Monte T. An interview with Dr. Anthony Sattilaro. *East-West Journal* (March 1981): 24–29.

Morishige F and Murata A. Prolongation of survival times in terminal human cancer by administration of supplemental ascorbate. *Journal of the International Academy of Preventive Medicine* 5 (1979): 47–52.

Moss R. *The Cancer Syndrome.* New York: Grove Press, 1980.

Moss R. *The Cancer Industry.* New York: Paragon Press, 1989.

Dr. Harold W. Manner: the man who cures cancer. *Mother Earth News* (November-December 1978): 17–24.

Andrew Saul: You can be your own doctor. *Mother Earth News* 85 (January-February 1984): 17–23.

Mothering Magazine. *Vaccinations: The Rest of the Story.* Chicago: Mothering Books, 1993.

Mowat F. *Never Cry Wolf.* New York: Dell, 1970.

Mullins E. *Murder by Injection; The Medical Conspiracy against America.* Staunton, VA: National Council for Medical Research, 1988.

Murata A. Virucidal activity of vitamin C: Vitamin C for the prevention and treatment of viral diseases. *Proceedings of the First Intersectional Congress of Microbiological Societies, Science Council of Japan* 3 (1975): 432–42.

Murata A, Morishige F, and Yamaguchi H. Prolongation of survival times of terminal cancer patients by administration of large doses of ascorbate. *International Journal of Vitamin and Nutrition Research Suppl.* 23 (1982): 103–113.

Murray F. *Program Your Heart for Health.* New York: Larchmont, 1978.

Murray M. *The Complete Book of Juicing.* Rocklin, CA: Prima Publishing, 1992.

Myers JA. The role of some nutritional elements in the health of the teeth and their supporting structures. *Annals of Dentistry* 22 (1958): 35–47.

Natenberg M. *The Legacy of Dr. Wiley.* Chicago: Regent House, 1957.

Natural vitamin E for heart diseases. *Popular Science Digest* (March 1953): 4–6.

Newmark HL. Stability of vitamin B_{12} in the presence of ascorbic acid. *American Journal of Clinical Nutrition* 29 (1976): 645–49.

Null G, et al. Vitamin C and the treatment of cancer: abstracts and commentary from the scientific literature. *The Townsend Letter for Doctors and Patients* (April-May 1997).

Osmond H and Hoffer A. Massive niacin treatment in schizophrenia: review of a nine-year study. *Lancet* 1 (1962): 316–19.

Parham B. *What's Wrong with Eating Meat?* Denver, CO: Ananda Marga, 1979.

Park CH. Biological nature of the effect of ascorbic acids on the growth of human leukemic cells. *Cancer Research* 45 (1985): 3969–973.

Passwater R. *Supernutrition.* New York: Dial, 1985.

Pauling L. Orthomolecular psychiatry. *Science* 160 (1968): 265–71.

Pauling L. *Vitamin C, the Common Cold, and the Flu.* San Francisco: W. H. Freeman, 1976.

Pauling L. Plowboy interview: Dr. Linus Pauling. *Mother Earth News* (January-February 1978): 17–22.

Pauling L. On good nutrition for the good life. *Executive Health* 17 (4 January 1981).

Pauling L. On vitamin C and infectious diseases. *Executive Health* 19 (4 January 1983): 1–5.

Pauling L. *How to Live Longer and Feel Better.* New York: W. H. Freeman, 1986.

Pauling L and Rath M. An orthomolecular theory of human health and disease. *Journal of Orthomolecular Medicine* 6 (1991): 135–138.

Pauling L, et al. Effect of dietary ascorbic acid on the incidence of spontaneous mammary tumors in RIII mice. *Proceedings of the National Academy of Sciences.* 82 (August 1985): 5185–189.

Pfeiffer CC. "Mental Illness and Schizophrenia." In *The Nutrition Connection.* New York: Thorsons, 1987.

Physician's Desk Reference. Montvale, New Jersey: Medical Economics Data Production Company, 1994.

Price W. *Nutrition and Physical Degeneration.* La Mesa, CA: Price-Pottenger Nutrition Foundation, 1970.

Prien EL and Gershoff SF. Magnesium oxide-pyridoxine therapy for recurrent calcium oxalate calculi. *J Urol* 112 (1974): 509–12.

Quigley DT. *The National Malnutrition.* Milwaukee, WI: Lee Foundation for Nutritional Research, 1948.

Raasch C and Cochran W. Millions injected into health care debate. *Democrat and Chronicle* [Rochester, New York]. (17 April 1994).

Ratcliff JD. For heart disease: vitamin E. *Coronet* (October 1948).

Rath M. *Eradicating Heart Disease.* San Francisco, CA: Health Now, 1993.

Rattan V, et al. Effect of combined supplementation of magnesium oxide and pyridoxine in calcium-oxalate stone formers. *Urol Res* 22 (1994): 161–165.

Ray O and Ksir C. *Drugs, Society, and Human Behavior,* 5th ed. Mosby, St. Louis: Times Mirror, 1990, 198.

Rehert I. Doctor finds cure in macrobiotic diet. *Los Angeles Times.* (13 December 1981).

Riker J. The Salk vaccine. *New Directions* (Summer 1991): 21–25.

Rimm EB, et al. Vitamin E consumption and the risk of coronary heart disease in men. *New England Journal of Medicine* 328 (1993): 1450–456.

Rinse J. Atherosclerosis: prevention and cure [parts 1 and 2]. *Prevention* (November/December 1975).

Rinse J. Cholesterol and phospholipids in relation to atherosclerosis. *American Laboratory Magazine* (April 1978).

Riordan HD. *Medical Mavericks.* Wichita, KS: Bio-Communications Press, c.1988.

Riordan HD, Jackson JA, and Neathery S. Vitamin, blood lead, and urine pyrrole levels in Down's syndrome. *American Clinical Laboratory* (January 1990): 8–9.

Riordan HD, Jackson JA, Schultz M. Case study: high-dose intravenous vitamin C in the treatment of a patient with adenocarcinoma of the kidney. *J Ortho Med* 5 (1990): 5–7.

Riordan NH, et al. Intravenous ascorbate as a tumor cytotoxic chemotherapeutic agent. *Medical Hypotheses* 44 (1995): 207–13.

Riordan N, Jackson JA, Riordan HD. Intravenous vitamin C in a terminal cancer patient. J Ortho Med 11(1996): 80–82.

Rivers JM. Safety of high-level vitamin C injection. In "Third Conference on Vitamin C," *Annals of the New York Academy of Sciences* 498 (1987): 95–102.

Robertson L, et al. *Laurel's Kitchen.* New York: Bantam, 1976.

Rodale JI. *The Healthy Hunzas.* Emmaus, PA: Rodale Press, 1948.

Rogers LL, Pelton RB, and Williams RJ. Voluntary alcohol consumption by rats following administration of glutamine. *J Biol Chem* 214 (1955): 503–06.

Rogoff JM, et al. Vitamin C and insulin action. *Pennsylvania Medical Journal* 47 (1944): 579–82.

Sabin AB. Vitamin C in relation to experimental poliomyelitis. *Journal of Experimental Medicine* 69 (1939): 507–15.

Sandler BP. Treatment of tuberculosis with a low carbohydrate, high protein diet. *Diseases of the Chest* 17 (1950): 398.

Saul AW. Plowboy interview: You can be your own doctor. *Mother Earth News* 85 (January-February 1984): 17–23.

Saul AW. *Paperback Clinic.* Seneca Falls, NY: New York Chiropractic College Press, 1994.

Scher J, et al. Massive vitamin C as an adjunct in methadone maintenance and detoxification of narcotic addicts. *Journal of Orthomolecular Psychiatry* 5 (1976): 191–198.

Schlegel JU, et al. The role of ascorbic acid in the prevention of bladder tumor formation. *J Urol* 103 (1970): 155.

Shafer CF. Ascorbic acid and atherosclerosis. *American Journal of Clinical Nutrition* 23 (1970): 27.

Shute E. Proposed study of vitamin E therapy. *Can Med Assoc J* 106 (May 1972): 1057.

Shute E. Vitamin E fatigue? [Letter.] *Calif Med* 119 (1973): 73.

Shute E. *The Vitamin E Story: The Medical Memoirs of Evan Shute.* Burlington, Ontario: Welch Publishing, 1985.

Shute E, et al. *The Heart and Vitamin E.* London, Canada: The Shute Foundation for Medical Research, 1963.

Shute WE. *Health Preserver.* Emmaus, PA: Rodale Press, 1977.

Shute WE. *The Vitamin E Book.* New Canaan, CT: Keats Publishing, 1978.

Shute WE. *Your Child and Vitamin E.* New Canaan, CT: Keats Publishing, 1979.

Shute WE and Taub HJ. *Vitamin E for Ailing and Healthy Hearts.* New York: Pyramid House, 1969.

Smith JL and Hodges RE. Serum levels of vitamin C in relation to dietary and supplemental intake of vitamin C in smokers and nonsmokers. In "Third Conference on Vitamin C," *Annals of the New York Academy of Sciences* 498 (1987).

Smith L, ed. *Clinical Guide to the Use of Vitamin C: The Clinical Experiences of Frederick R. Klenner, M.D.* Tacoma, WA: Life Sciences Press, 1988.

Smith SF and Smith CM. *Personal Health Choices.* Boston: Jones and Bartlett, 1990.

Solomon J. Placebo revisited: An update on a very useful agent. *Consultant* (December 1982): 220–29.

Spittle CR. Atherosclerosis and vitamin C. *Lancet* 2 (1971): 1280–281.

Spittle CR. The action of vitamin C on blood vessels. *American Heart Journal* 88 (1974): 387–88.

Spock B. *Baby and Child Care.* New York: Pocket Books, 1976.

Stampfer MJ, et al. Vitamin E consumption and the risk of coronary disease in women. *New England Journal of Medicine* 328 (1993): 1444–449.

Stahelin HB, et al. Vitamin C levels lower in cancer group. *J Nat Canc Inst* 73 (1984): 1463–468.

Stoll W. *Saving Yourself from the Disease-Care Crisis.* Panama City, FL: [Self-published], 1996.

Stone I. *The Healing Factor.* New York: Putnam, 1972.

Straus H. *Dr. Max Gerson: Healing the Hopeless.* With Barbara Marinacci. Kingston, Ontario: Quarry Press, 2002.

Sugiura K. On the relation of diets to the development, prevention, and treatment of cancer, with special reference to cancer of the stomach and liver. *Journal of Nutrition* 44 (1951): 345.

Taub HJ. *Keeping Healthy in a Polluted World.* New York: Penguin, 1975.

Torch WC. Diphtheria-pertussis-tetanus (DPT) immunization: A potential cause of the sudden infant death syndrome (SIDS). [Abstract.] *Neurology* 32 (1982): A169.

Torch WC. Characteristics of diphtheria-pertussis-tetanus (DPT) postvaccinal deaths and DPT-caused sudden infant death syndrome (SIDS): A review. [Abstract.] *Neurology* Suppl. 1 (1986): 148.

Tsao CS, Dunham WB, and Ping YL. In vivo antineoplastic activity of ascorbic acid for human mammary tumor. *In Vivo* 2 (1988): 147–150.

Turner J. *The Chemical Feast.* New York: Grossman, 1970.

Verlangieri AJ. *The Role of Vitamin C in Diabetic and Non-diabetic Atherosclerosis.* Bulletin, Vol. 21. University of Mississippi: Bureau of Pharm. Services, 1985.

Wachowicz K. Cancer victim endorses raw foods, sprout therapy. *The Colonian* [Albany, NY] (16 November 1981).

Waldbott GL, Burgstahler AW, and McKinney HL. *Fluoridation: The Great Dilemma.* Lawrence, KS: Coronado Press, 1978.

Walker AM, et al. Diphtheria-tetanus-pertussis immunization and sudden infant death syndrome. *Am Jour Pub Health* 77 (1987): 945–51.

Walker M. *Dirty Medicine: Science, Big Business, and the Assault on Natural Health Care.* London: Slingshot Publications, 1993.

Walker NW. *Diet and Salad Suggestions.* Phoenix, AZ: Norwalk Press, 1971.

Wapnick AA. The effect of ascorbic acid deficiency on desferrioxamine-induced urinary iron excretion. *British Journal of Haematology* 17 (1969): 563–68.

Warmbrand M. *Encyclopedia of Health and Nutrition.* New York: Pyramid, 1962.

Werbach M. *Nutritional Influences on Illness.* New Canaan, CT: Keats Publishing, 1988.

Werbach M. *Textbook of Nutritional Medicine.* Tarzana, CA: Third Line Press, 1999.

Whitaker J. Act now to protect your health. *Health and Healing Newsletter* Suppl. (September 1993): 1–4.

White K. PACs on precise missions. *Democrat and Chronicle* [Rochester, NY] (6 March 1994).

Wigmore A. *Why Suffer?* New York: Hemisphere Press, 1964.

Wigmore A. *Recipes for Longer Life.* Garden City Park, NY: Avery, 1982.

Wigmore A. *Be Your Own Doctor.* Garden City Park, NY: Avery, 1983.

Wilcox A, Weinberg C, and Baird D. Caffeinated beverages and decreased fertility. *The Lancet* 8626-7 (December 1988): 1473–476.

Wiley HW. *The History of a Crime Against the Food Law.* Washington, D.C.: [Self-published] 1929. Reprinted Milwaukee, WI: Lee Foundation for Nutritional Research, 1955.

Williams RJ. *Nutrition and Alcoholism.* Norman, OK: University of Oklahoma Press, 1951.

Williams RJ. *Biochemical Individuality: The Basis for the Genetotrophic Concept.* New York: Wiley, 1956. Reprinted Austin, TX: University of Texas Press, 1973.

Williams RJ. *Alcoholism: The Nutritional Approach.* Austin, TX: University of Texas Press, 1959.

Williams RJ. *Nutrition in a Nutshell.* New York: Dolphin Books, 1962.

Williams RJ. *You Are Extraordinary.* New York: Random House, 1967.

Williams RJ. *Nutrition Against Disease.* New York: Pitman, 1971.

Williams RJ. Biochemical individuality: A story of neglect. *Journal of the International Academy of Preventive Medicine* 1 (1974): 99–106.

Williams RJ. The neglect of nutritional science in cancer research. *Congressional Record* (16 October 1974): S.19204.

Williams RJ. *Physicians' Handbook of Nutritional Science.* Springfield, IL: Charles C. Thomas, 1975.

Williams RJ. *The Prevention of Alcoholism through Nutrition.* New York: Bantam, 1981.

Williams RJ and Kalita DK, eds. *A Physician's Handbook on Orthomolecular Medicine.* New Canaan, CT: Keats Publishing, 1977.

Williams SR. *Nutrition and Diet Therapy,* 7th edition. St. Louis: Mosby, 1993.

Willis GC. The reversibility of atherosclerosis. *Canadian Medical Association Journal of Nutrition* 77 (1957): 106–109.

Winacour J, ed. *The Story of the Titanic as Told by Its Survivors.* New York: Dover, 1960.

Yiamouyiannis J. *Fluoride: The Aging Factor.* Delaware, OH: Health Action Press 1986.

Yonemoto RH, et al. Enhanced lymphocyte blastogenesis by oral ascorbic acid. *Proceedings of the American Association for Cancer Research* 17 (1976): 288.

Yuan JM, et al. Diet and breast cancer in Shanghai and Tianjin, China. *British Journal of Cancer* 71 (1995): 1353–358.

Zannoni VG, et al. Ascorbic acid, alcohol, and environmental chemicals. In "Third Conference on Vitamin C," *Annals of the New York Academy of Sciences* 498: (1987).

Zuskin E, Lewis AJ, Bouhuys A. Inhibition of histamine-induced airway constriction by ascorbic acid. *Journal of Allergy and Clinical Immunology* 51 (1973): 218–26.

Index

migraines, p 65

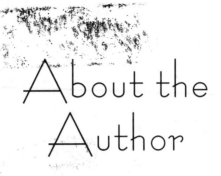

About the Author

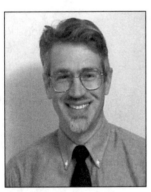

Andrew Saul, Ph.D., a biologist and teacher by training, has been a consulting specialist in natural healing for more than twenty-five years, helping medical doctors' problem patients to get better. He has taught hundreds of students at New York Chiropractic College and the State University of New York. Dr. Saul's previous book, *Paperback Clinic,* has been used as both a college textbook and reference work for health practitioners. Dr. Saul is also the author of *Fire Your Doctor!* (Basic Health Publications, 2005). He lives and practices in Upstate New York.